Lisa Simpson

Lecture Notes
the Liver

# Lecture Notes on the Liver

Richard Thompson

DM, FRCP
Consultant Physician
St Thomas' Hospital
London

BLACKWELL

SCIENTIFIC PUBLICATIONS

OXFORD LONDON EDINBURGH
BOSTON PALO ALTO MELBOURNE

©1985 by
Blackwell Scientific Publications
Editorial offices:
Osney Mead, Oxford, OX2 0EL
8 John Street, London, WC1N 2ES
23 Ainslie Place, Edinburgh, EH3 6AJ
52 Beacon Street, Boston
Massachusetts 02108, USA
667 Lytton Avenue, Palo Alto
California 94301, USA
107 Barry Street, Carlton
Victoria 3053, Australia

All rights reserved. No part of this
publication may be reproduced, stored
in a retrieval system, or transmitted,
in any form or by any means,
electronic, mechanical, photocopying,
recording or otherwise without the
prior permission of the copyright
owner

First published 1985

Set by Mayhew Typesetting, Bristol
Printed and bound by
Billing & Sons Ltd, Worcester

DISTRIBUTORS

USA
Blackwell Mosby book Distributors
11830 Westline Industrial Drive
St Louis, Missouri 63141

Canada
Blackwell Mosby Book
Distributors
120 Melford Drive, Scarborough
Ontario M1B 2X4

Australia
Blackwell Scientific Publications
(Australia) Pty Ltd
107 Barry Street
Carlton, Victoria 3053

British Library
Cataloguing in Publication Data

Thompson, Richard P.H.
Lecture notes on the liver.
1. Liver — Diseases
I. Title
616.3'62      RC845

ISBN 0-632-01338-9

# Contents

Preface, vii

1 Symptoms and Signs of Liver and Biliary Disease, 1

2 Pathophysiology and Treatment of Complications, 13

3 Investigations, 49

4 Hyperbilirubinaemia and Jaundice, 68

5 Acute Viral Hepatitis, 79

6 Bacterial and Parasitic Infections, 93

7 Drug and Toxic Hepatitis, 103

8 Chronic Hepatitis, 111

9 Alcoholic Disease, 119

10 Cirrhosis, 126

11 Tumours, 139

12 Vascular Disorders, 143

13 Infiltration and Metabolic Disorders, 146

14 Pregnancy, 152

15 Bowel Disease, 154

16 Gall Stones, 156

vi  *Contents*

17 Tumours of the Biliary Tract, 164

18 Congenital and Other Lesions of the Biliary Tract, 170

General Reading, 173

Index, 174

# Preface

This latest book in the Lecture Notes series is aimed chiefly at the undergraduate medical student, though the postgraduate may also find it useful.

The pathophysiology and diseases of the liver and its biliary tract are in many ways quite separate from those of the gastro-intestinal tract and represent too large a subject to be covered adequately by books on general gastroenterology, and therefore, I believe, merit their own Lecture Notes.

Apart from the classic diseases such as virus hepatitis and cirrhosis, I have also described how the liver may be affected in non-hepatic disorders such as pregnancy and inflammatory bowel disease. Diseases of the liver are not as common as, for instance, those of the stomach and bowel, but they do cause difficulties in diagnoses and, I believe, play a significant role in examinations!

I have included a list of general texts for further reading and, at the end of each chapter, some modern reviews which I hope the reader may find useful.

I shall look forward to receiving comments, be they favourable or critical.

*R.P.H. Thompson*

# Chapter 1
# Symptoms and Signs of Liver and Biliary Disease

## SYMPTOMS

The symptoms of liver disease are often non-specific, e.g. anorexia, lassitude and nausea. Loss of weight may be disguised by fluid retention, i.e. oedema and ascites. And while anorexia and lack of desire to smoke are often prominent in hepatitis, they are also suffered by any patient who is jaundiced of whatever cause. Excessive tiredness and sleepiness and inappropriate behaviour develop in severe liver disease with hepatic encephalopathy (*see* chapter 2). This is noticed by relatives or the doctor rather than by the patient.

### Pain

Frequently liver disease is painless. Pain, however, from the liver is felt in the right hypochondrium, and over the right lower ribs radiating round to the back.

In certain cases pain will be associated with liver disease. Acute hepatitis causes the liver to swell and ache. Pain from primary or secondary carcinoma of the liver may make the last weeks of a patient's life miserable, the pain often being worse on breathing and coughing, similar to true pleural pain. A dragging feeling in the abdomen may come from an enlarged liver or spleen and the patient may describe his or her abdominal muscles as tight.

Some gall stones cause no pain, but most eventually do so. Biliary colic typically comes in bouts. While present it is fairly constant in the right hypochondrium, with less of the great variation in intensity seen in the gripes of intestinal colic. More chronic, dull, right hypochrondrial and back pain can occur with stones in the gallbladder, *chronic cholecystitis*. Gall stone pain, however, is also often felt in the epigastrium, but much less commonly elsewhere in the abdomen. A severe, acute pain occurs over the acutely inflammed gallbladder *acute cholecystitis* (*see* chapter 16).

1

2    *Chapter 1*

## Jaundice

Jaundice is a symptom usually first noticed by the patient's relatives or doctor. It is eventually noticed by the patient through the discolouration of his or her eyes. If there is conjugated hyperbilirubinaemia (*see* chapter 2), dark urine and pale stools will be noticed before the jaundice.

## Itching

Itching commonly occurs with both extrahepatic or intrahepatic cholestasis (*see* chapter 2) and its presence does not help to differentiate between them.

## Bleeding

Haematemesis and melaena due to bleeding from the upper gastrointestinal tract occurs in severe liver disease, often when there is portal hypertension. It can be profuse. Easy bruising may also be noticed.

## Other features

Amenorrhoea, loss of libido and impotence are frequent in chronic liver disease. Alcohol will cause them before cirrhosis develops. Swelling of the ankles due to oedema can be the first symptom of cirrhosis.

## Alcohol intake

Frequently played down or denied by the patient, persistent tactful questioning about alcohol intake may be needed to elicit a more accurate account! 'Double what the patient says and halve what his wife says' is sometimes true, but often the wife conives with her spouse. Check through the main types of drink such as beer, wine, spirits, sherry etc. Suggest a large amount ('Half a bottle of sherry a day?') and watch the patient's response. Does he or she drink regularly at lunch?

### Past history of jaundice

Recurrent attacks of jaundice suggest gall stones, previous biliary surgery, alcoholic liver disease, chronic hepatitis or, rarely, a familial jaundice.

*Symptoms and Signs of Liver and Biliary Disease* 3

**Parenteral transfer of virus hepatitis**

Has there been past administration of blood, plasma, or blood products (e.g. clotting factor concentrates), injections, either medical, especially when they are given abroad, or from drug abuse, tattooing etc.?

**Drug history**

Since many drugs can on occasions idiosyncratically damage the liver (*see* chapter 7), a careful note must be made of all drugs taken by the patient. If necessary check with the patients' GP, for some patients have forgotten, or do not know, what they have received. Check the complete composition of tablets as their constituents are sometimes surprising.

**Travel abroad**

Viral hepatitis (*see* chapter 5) is more common in warmer countries. Some tropical diseases involve the liver (*see* chapter 6).

**Surgical history**

Liver disease can follow perfect or imperfect biliary surgery. There may be ascending cholangitis (*see* chapter 16), or a liver abscess (*see* chapter 6) may develop some years after an abdominal operation.

**PATIENT'S HISTORY**

The patient should be carefully asked about:
    alcohol intake
    past history of jaundice
    past history of transfusions, injections
    drug history
    travel history
    past history of surgery

**GENERAL EXAMINATION**

Certain physical signs are particularly associated with liver disease (Figure 1.1).

4  Chapter 1

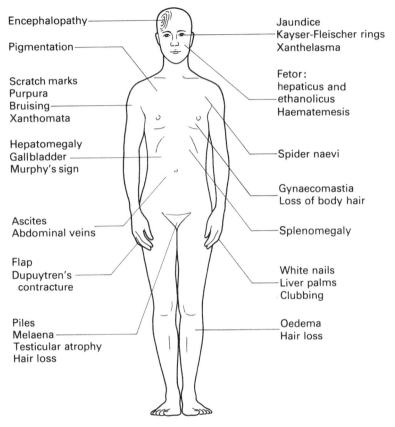

**Fig. 1.1** Physical signs of a patient with liver and biliary disease.

## Hands and arms

### LIVER PALMS

Erythema, liver palms, of the thenar and hypothenar areas of the palm, and sometimes of the finger pulps, and of the soles of the feet, is traditionally associated with cirrhosis. However, it also develops in other non-hepatic chronic debilitating disease, e.g. rheumatoid arthritis, and in pregnancy.

*Symptoms and Signs of Liver and Biliary Disease*     5

## WHITE NAILS

Loss of the lunulae, so that the nails become uniformly white, is associated with liver disease, but is not specific for liver disease.

## FINGER CLUBBING

Clubbing of the fingers is not common in liver disease, but can be seen in long-standing primary biliary and cryptogenic cirrhosis (*see* chaptér 10).

## DUPUYTREN'S CONTRACTURE

Thickening and contracture of the fascia on the ulnar side of the palm and fixed flexion of the medial fingers occurs more frequently in alcoholics with or without cirrhosis than in normal people. It is also more common in epileptics.

## SCRATCHES

Scratch marks are seen in patients with itching.

## MUSCLE WASTING

Wasting of muscles is common in the alcoholic.

## LIVER FLAP

A coarse, jerky, inconstant, flapping tremor of the outstretched hands, (*asterixis*) is a sign of hepatic encephalopathy, and therefore of severe liver disease, but also occurs in renal failure and other severe metabolic disorders.

To demonstrate asterixis, ask the patient to hold his or her arms out for 60 seconds with the fingers spread, the wrists dorsiflexed and eyes closed. A fine, more regular tremor of the hands is common in alcoholics.

## PERIPHERAL NEUROPATHY

The alcoholic's hands and feet are typically cold and sweating, due to autonomic neuropathy. A lack of peripheral hair on the arms and legs may also be noted. Objective signs of a peripheral motor and sensory neuropathy may be present, but subjective paraesthesiae without signs are more common.

6 *Chapter 1*

## Head and neck

### ENCEPHALOPATHY

Difficult to detect, encephalopathy varies from a dulling and slowing of the wits with increased sleepiness to stupor and deep coma. In the early stages a history from relatives is more informative. Later the patient becomes persistently drowsy, sometimes with periods of delirium and violence, and finally comatose (hepatic coma). Hyperventilation is seen. The degrees of classification of encephalopathy are given in Table 1.1.

**Table 1.1** Stages of hepatic encephalopathy.

| | | Stages | |
|---|---|---|---|
| 1 | 2 | 3 | 4 |
| Euphoria or depression | Drowsiness | Stupor | Coma |
| Slow thoughts | Loss of sphincter control | Confusion | Decreasing response to stimuli |
| Disordered sleep Slight flap | Flap | Rousable | |

### DELIRIUM TREMENS

Due to alcoholism (*see* chapter 9), *delirium tremens* may vary from the frequently seen anxiety, tremulousness, and tremor of the hands and head of the heavy drinker, to terrifying hallucinations, confusion and delirium. This usually develops in the alcoholic when alcohol is withdrawn, and frequently there is underlying chronic liver disease.

### FITS

Epileptic fits ('rum fits') may follow alcohol withdrawal, or be due to hypoglycaemia during a 'binge'. They also occur in coma due to severe liver failure.

# Symptoms and Signs of Liver and Biliary Disease

## FETOR

Hepatic fetor is a musty smell to the breath in patients with hepatic encephalopathy, but is not easy to detect. Alcoholic fetor is much commoner!

## FASCIES

The alcoholic's face is often diagnostic. Initially it is obese, flushed and sweating, with fine, dilated, bright-red, tortuous vessels on the cheeks (paper money skin) and conjunctivae (blood-shot). These appearances are often the only clue to excessive alcohol intake, even if it is denied.

## SPIDER NAEVI

Large, bright-red telangiectases with a central arteriole dividing horizontally in the skin into fine radiating 'legs' are known as spider naevi. The arteriole or 'body' may be raised (*papular*), and the whole naevus can be blanched by pressure on this central body with an orange stick or pencil. For some reason they are found predominantly on the cheeks, neck and shoulders. One or two 'spiders' may be found in normal people, but more suggest chronic liver disease, usually alcoholic cirrhosis. They also temporarily increase in size and number during normal pregnancy.

## PAROTID ENLARGEMENT

Parotid enlargement is unusual in the UK, but develops in a few alcoholics, particularly in North America.

## MUCOSAE CYANOSIS

Central cyanosis of the mucosae occasionally occurs in chronic liver disease, usually accompanied by clubbing, and is due to arteriovenous shunting of blood in the lungs.

## BRUISING

Bruising either spontaneous or at the sites of trauma or venepuncture, occurs in patients with liver disease and abnormal coagulation of the blood (*see* chapter 2).

8     *Chapter 1*

## PIGMENTATION

Pigmentation of the skin progressively develops in primary biliary cirrhosis and to a lesser extent in haemochromatosis.

## XANTHOMATA

Deposits of cholesterol esters in the eyelids, *xanthelasma*, palms or skin of the neck are seen in patients with prolonged cholestasis, usually primary biliary cirrhosis (*see* chapter 10).

## KAYSER-FLEISCHER RINGS

Indistinct brown rings around the edge of the cornea, Kayser-Fleischer rings, are seen in patients with Wilson's disease (*see* chapter 10). They are due to deposits of copper on the back of the cornea. They are best seen with the ophthalmologist's slit-lamp, but are often visible just with a torch, if carefully looked for.

## JAUNDICE

Jaundice is not easily detected in the sclera until the bilirubin level in blood reaches 30 $\mu$mol/litre (2 mg/100 ml). Even then it is easily missed, especially in artificial light. It is looked for by gently pulling down the lower lid with the thumb to expose more sclera. As jaundice increases, the skin and palate also become yellow.

### Chest and abdomen

Certain physical signs concentrating on the chest and abdomen area are characteristic of a patient with liver and biliary disease (Figure 1.2).

## OBESITY

Obesity of the trunk is a feature of alcoholism.

## GYNAECOMASTIA

Gynaecomastia occurs in men with chronic liver disease, but is more often a side effect of treatment with spironolactone.

# Symptoms and Signs of Liver and Biliary Disease

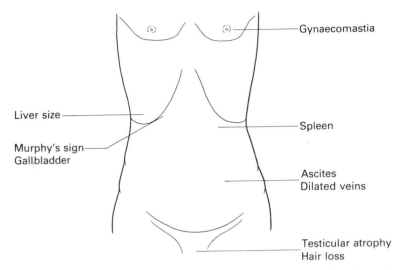

**Fig. 1.2** Physical signs concentrating on the chest and abdomen of a patient with liver and biliary disease.

## TESTICULAR ATROPHY

Difficult to assess accurately, testicular atrophy also occurs in patients with chronic liver disease, as does loss of pubic hair.

## ABDOMINAL WALL VEINS

Enlarged abdominal wall veins may be seen in patients with ascites and portal hypertension, or with blockage of the inferior vena cava. Ascites and, more dramatically, blockage of the cava, impair the flow of blood up the cava and so blood passes instead up the collateral vessels in the anterior abdominal wall. In this case a finger placed on a vein will cause the segment of vein above it to collapse, as Harvey showed, i.e. the blood is flowing upwards.

Occasionally, if the umbilical vein is patent and there is intrahepatic portal hypertension (*see* chapter 2), pressure is transmitted from the left portal vein to the veins around the umbilicus, which dilate. Mostly there are only one or two swollen veins, but occasionally a leash of vessels draining away from the umbilicus develops. This is the rare *caput medusae*.

10 *Chapter 1*

## LIVER

It is often believed that the diseased liver is always enlarged, but this is not so. Particularly large livers develop when they are infiltrated by primary or secondary carcinomata, and in biliary cirrhosis. The lower edge may feel knobbly, but this is not always easy to detect.

A small liver often, but not always, occurs in end-stage cirrhosis, particularly in the alcoholic, and the liver also rapidly shrinks in acute hepatic necrosis as the liver cells die and the reticulin framework collapses.

Liver size is assessed by inspection, palpation, percussion and by auscultation. Inspection may reveal a fullness in the right hypochondrium if the patient is thin. Palpate the lower edge of the liver with the hand held flat on the abdomen and parallel with the edge of the ribs. Ask the patient to breathe deeply so as to move the edge during inspiration on to your hand, and note any tenderness or irregularity. Once an edge has been located, follow it across to the left costal margin, and to the right flank. Note that an enlarged left lobe can be difficult to distinguish from an enlarged spleen, and that sometimes a soft normal right lobe extends down into the right flank (Riedel's lobe).

Next percuss the area of liver dullness over the lower right ribs keeping the passive finger in the coronal plane. This will approximately indicate the size of the liver from top to bottom, but the upper border is particularly difficult to percuss accurately.

Auscultate for a vascular bruit while the patient stops breathing, and for a rub while breathing.

Try the tickling test for liver size. Place the diaphragm of the stethoscope over the right lower ribs and tickle the right abdominal skin upwards towards it with the finger. The sound suddenly becomes louder when the lower edge of the liver is crossed, but the finger must not be nearer than 3 cm from the stethoscope.

## SPLEEN

Spleens are often difficult to feel, sometimes because too much pressure with the hand pushes it away. Spleen tips are best detected at the peak of inspiration when they descend on to the fingers as the diaphragm moves.

Reach over the patient and place the left hand over the lower left ribs with the thumb on the costal edge. Place the right hand almost parallel to the costal margin and gently press as the patient breathes in. The spleen tip is often soft, sometimes tender, and may slip over the fingers. The position of the left thumb avoids mistaking a mobile costal cartilage for the spleen. If still no spleen, turn the patient half on his or her right side towards you

*Symptoms and Signs of Liver and Biliary Disease* 11

and try again. Try again the next day.

Large spleens enlarge down towards the pubis. They are easily felt as a firm mass, and a notch can sometimes be felt on the medial border. A large left lobe of the liver can mimic a moderately enlarged spleen, as also less often can an enlarged left kidney.

Percussion of the lower left ribs along the midaxillary line is usually dull when the spleen is large, but this sign is unreliable.

Occasionally a rub can be auscultated over the spleen over a splenic infarct.

Splenomegaly frequently occurs in chronic liver disease when there is portal hypertension, but the degree of enlargement is surprisingly not related to the severity of portal hypertension, nor to the risk of bleeding from varices. The spleen may also enlarge during acute viral hepatitis, particularly when this is due to glandular fever, and when the portal vein is blocked by thrombosis or tumour.

## GALLBLADDER

An enlarged gallbladder is difficult to feel, but may become palpable when the patient rolls half on his or her left side away from the examiner.

Courvoisier's law, namely that an enlarged palpable gallbladder suggests a carcinoma of pancreas rather than gall stones, is statistically correct but unreliable (*see* chapter 16).

## ASCITES

Probably at least a litre of ascites is needed in order to be detected clinically. The ascitic abdomen sags backwards in the flanks when the patient lies supine, and hangs forward when he or she stands. Place the hands between the flanks and the mattress and feel whether they seem to be full of fluid.

Percuss the flanks. These should be dull if there is ascites with the anterior abdomen resonant as the air-filled bowel floats forwards. Then roll the patient on one side and percuss the upper flank. If the ascites is not tense the upper flank becomes resonant as the fluid falls downwards to the lowerside and the bowel floats upwards.

Flicking one flank to see if a percussion wave can be felt in the other flank is an unreliable sign of ascites.

Probably the most reliable means of detecting ascites is to insert a fine needle into a flank with the patient supine, and aspirate. There is no risk of perforating the bowel as long as it is not obstructed. Ultrasonography is an expensive way of confirming it.

Ascites develops in patients with chronic liver disease and portal

12 *Chapter 1*

hypertension, in cases of severe acute hepatitis, and in malignancy or intra-abdominal tuberculosis when the peritoneum is involved by seedling metastases or tubercles.

## HAEMORRHOIDS

Haemorrhoids (piles) may rarely be caused by portal hypertension, but are more usually unrelated.

## Legs

### OEDEMA

Pitting oedema is common in chronic liver disease, and precedes ascites. It can extend up the legs to the sacrum, scrotum and abdominal wall.

### PERIPHERAL NEUROPATHY

Loss of hair, and cold, sweating feet are common in the alcoholic.

### CLUBBING

Clubbing of the toes and erythema of the soles are similar but less marked to changes in the hands. Bruising and scratch marks may also be seen in the legs.

### MUSCLE WASTING

Wasting of the muscles of the limbs is another feature of the alcoholic.

## FURTHER READING

McFarlane I.G. (1984) Autoimmunity in liver disease. *Clinical Science* **67**, 569–78.
Sherlock S. & Summerfield J.A. (1979). *A Colour Atlas of Liver Disease*. Wolfe, London.
Thompson R.P.H. (1980) *An Introduction to Physical Signs*. Blackwell Scientific Publications, Oxford.

# Chapter 2
# Pathophysiology and Treatment
# of Complications

There are many aspects of abnormal function of the liver and other organs in the patient with liver disease, and they are described individually in this chapter. Some are first grouped under the term liver cell failure.

## LIVER CELL FAILURE

Failure of the normal function of hepatic parenchymal cells results in biochemical changes, such as jaundice, abnormal clotting and low serum albumin levels, and finally encephalopathy. It is analogous to renal failure producing uraemia. However, the vascular changes of portal hypertension will be discussed later in the chapter.

### Bilirubin metabolism

#### SYNTHESIS OF BILIRUBIN

All haem in the body is broken down to bilirubin, which is normally excreted solely by the liver into bile. The major source of bilirubin (80%) is the haem of haemoglobin in red blood cells (Figure 2.1), but some 15–20% derives from the breakdown of haem in enzymes, such as cytochromes, and in the liver. A small amount also comes from the premature breakdown of immature red cells in the bone marrow, so-called ineffective erythropoiesis.

Red blood cells are removed from blood by reticuloendothelial cells, particularly by those lining the blood vessels of the spleen and liver, but also by macrophages in other tissues, such as occurs in a bruise. Within these cells the iron is removed from the haem molecule, and its porphyrin ring selectively opened up at one site (at the $\alpha$ bridge) by the enzyme haem oxygenase (Figure 2.2). During this reaction carbon monoxide is released, the only reaction in the body to do so, and excreted in breath.

The product is biliverdin, which is then reduced to bilirubin by the enzyme biliverdin reductase. Almost all the biliverdin and bilirubin that are formed are specifically the $IX\alpha$ isomers, and there are only trace amounts of the other possible isomers that would be formed by splitting the porphyrin ring randomly at the other bridges.

14    Chapter 2

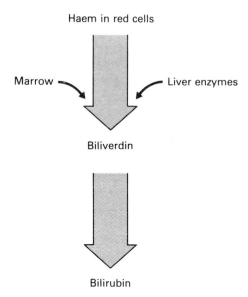

**Fig. 2.1**   Sources of haem converted to bilirubin.

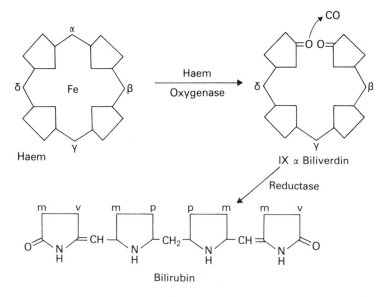

**Fig. 2.2**   Pathway of conversion of haem to bilirubin.

## CONJUGATION OF BILIRUBIN

The IXα bilirubin isomer, because of the relation of its rings and side chains (methyl, propyl and vinyl m, p, and v in Figure 2.2), takes up a complex three-dimensional conformation or shape, and is not the simple straight chain as shown in this figure. This shape gives special problems, rendering the molecule insoluble in water and difficult to excrete into bile without being further metabolised.

IXα bilirubin being soluble in fat or lipid, is carried from the reticuloendothelial cells, where it is formed, firmly bound to albumin in the blood. It is extracted from blood by the liver cells which leave the carrier albumin protein behind; an impressive, but little understood performance (Figure 2.3). That portion of bilirubin derived from hepatic haem enzymes presumably joins the rest directly in the liver cells.

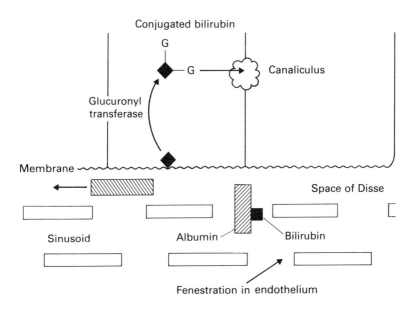

**Fig. 2.3** Scheme of uptake of bilirubin from the blood, conjugation by glucuronyltransferase in liver cells and excretion of conjugated bilirubin into the bile canaliculus.

Within the liver cells the bilirubin may be bound to carrier proteins. It is chiefly conjugated with one or two molecules of glururonic acid to give bilirubin monoglucuronides and diglucuronides by the enzyme glucuronyl

16                    *Chapter 2*

transferase, which is located on the membrane of the endoplasmic reticulum. The bilirubin glucuronides are then excreted into the bile canaliculi. In humans about 10% of bilirubin is also conjugated with other sugars such as glucose and xylose.

Bilirubin sugar conjugates are collectively called *conjugated bilirubin*. They are different in physical form and physiological properties from unconjugated bilirubin, for they are linear molecules, fully water soluble, and are readily excreted into bile. It is interesting what large changes in the physical properties such a small chemical change can produce.

This mechanism of alteration of molecules prior to excretion is common to the metabolism of many drugs in the liver.

## UROBILINOGEN

In bile, conjugated bilirubin is incorporated into bile acid micelles. It passes down the intestine with little being absorbed, and in the colon bacteria deconjugate and reduce it to various colourless compounds, the stercobilinogens or urobilinogens, which are chiefly excreted into the faeces. Oxidation of these to the brown urobilins and stercobilins gives the colour to normal faeces.

Some of the sterocobilinogens or urobilinogens are absorbed from the colon into portal venous blood, extracted from it by the liver and re-excreted into bile, thus undergoing an *enterohepatic circulation* (Figure 2.4). A small amount, however, escapes hepatic removal from portal blood, and passing through the liver into the systemic circulation is excreted by the kidney into urine.

The tests for detecting urobilinogen in urine are described in chapter 3.

## UNCONJUGATED VERSUS CONJUGATED BILIRUBIN

Free, unconjugated bilirubin, being lipid soluble, diffuses across cell membranes, so a small amount can be excreted directly across the bowel wall, *exsorption*.

It may also diffuse into the brain, particularly into the basal ganglia of neonates and cause kernicterus (*see* chapter 4). This is due to a combination of factors:

**1.** There is an extra load of bilirubin presented to the liver due to rapid haemolysis before and soon after birth.

**2.** The hepatic conjugation of bilirubin is particularly immature.

**3.** There is hypoxia and acidosis, which displace bilirubin from albumin into tissues.

**4.** Drugs such as salicylates and sulphonamides, if they are given, compete with bilirubin for albumin binding sites.

## Pathophysiology and Treatment of Complications

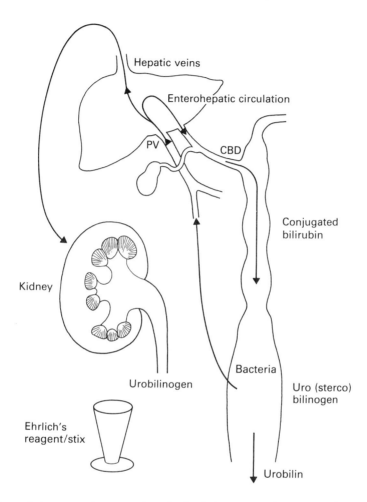

**Figure 2.4** Formation, enterohepatic circulation and renal excretion of urobilinogen.

Thus the premature baby with rhesus incompatibility is particularly liable to this irreversible brain damage.

Kernicterus does not occur in later life however severe the jaundice, as bilirubin is better conjugated.

Unconjugated bilirubin does not cross the renal glomerular membrane into urine since it is too firmly bound to albumin in blood. Jaundice due to unconjugated bilirubin in blood is therefore *acholuric*, that is without 'bile', or more correctly bilirubin, in the urine.

18                     *Chapter 2*

Conjugated bilirubin, however, can pass the glomeruli into urine. If renal function is normal, even in patients with complete obstruction of the biliary tree the bilirubin level in blood does not rise above about 800 $\mu$mol/litre (40 mg/100 ml) for the urinary leak of bilirubin acts as a safety valve (Table 2.1).

The chemical methods to measure unconjugated and conjugated bilirubin in blood are described in chapter 3.

**Table 2.1**   Features of unconjugated and conjugated bilirubin

|  | Unconjugated bilirubin | Conjugated bilirubin |
| --- | --- | --- |
| Solubility | Lipid | Water |
| Diazo reaction | Indirect | Direct |
| Urinary excretion | No (acholuria) | Yes |
| Biliary excretion | Trace | Yes |

### Formation of bile

Almost 1000–1500 ml of bile are secreted each day into the biliary canaliculi and small bile ducts. Since it can be secreted at a pressure greater than the hydrostatic pressure of blood, it cannot simply be a filtrate of plasma but must involve an energy mediated transport process. This is presumably in the biliary canaliculus, because microscopy reveals here a complex surface with microvilli characteristic of other secreting or absorbing membranes, such as the intestine. The canaliculus is too small for micropuncture, being simply an invagination between the adjoining membranes of two liver cells, so evidence on the initial formation of bile has to be indirect.

There are four major constituents of bile, namely: bile acids, the phospholipid lecithin (phosphatidylcholine), cholesterol and conjugated bilirubin; plus electrolytes, water and countless substances being excreted, such as urobilinogen and many drugs.

A major part of the fluid of bile is excreted in association with the energy-dependent transport of sodium, the so-called 'bile acid independent fraction', while another part is linked to the secretion of bile acids. Thus, bile acids are choleretic, or, in other words, when they are infused intravenously bile flow increases.

Bile acids spontaneously form tiny aggregates in solution called micelles

## Pathophysiology and Treatment of Complications 19

(see p. 22) that take up cholesterol and lecithin. It is not known whether these are initially formed in bile or whether some are preformed from tiny pieces of the canalicular membrane, complete with cholesterol and lecithin. If micelles are present in the canaliculus, then it is likely that lipid soluble substances will cross the canalicular membrane from liver cells and enter the micelles in bile. This would maintain a low effective concentration of these substances in bile outside the micelles, and so encourage then to pass without energy expenditure down a concentration gradient into bile — the so-called micellar 'sink'.

Electrolytes, water and mucus are added as bile passes down through larger bile ducts.

During fasting the majority of bile enters the gallbladder where it is concentrated, that is sodium and water are removed and the concentrations of bile acids, cholesterol etc., therefore rise. Some bile, however, always continues to flow past the cystic duct down to the intestine.

At the beginning of a meal the amino acids in food stimulate the duodenum to secrete into blood the hormone cholecystokinin (pancreozymin), which then causes the muscle of the gallbladder to contract and squeeze its stored bile into the intestine. In addition, the hormone secretin probably increases the secretion of sodium and water via the biliary tract into bile. Bile acids return from the intestine via portal venous blood in an enterohepatic circulation (see p. 21), are re-excreted by the liver, and increase the production of micellar bile until, some time after the meal is finished, they are again chiefly sequestered away in the gallbladder and bile flow once more falls.

## CHOLESTASIS

Stagnation of bile, or an obstruction of the flow of bile anywhere from the canaliculus to the papilla of Vater is known as *cholestasis*. It is a better and less confusing term than 'obstructive' jaundice which wrongly implies extrahepatic obstruction. Cholestasis, however, includes both intrahepatic causes such as hepatitis, as well as extrahepatic causes, such as gall stones.

The mechanism of cholestasis is obvious with extrahepatic lesions or intrahepatic space occupying lesions pressing on the main bile ducts, but it is not clear for other intrahepatic causes. Most diseases of the liver cells predominantly affect the secretion of substances into bile, rather than their metabolism within the cell. This is confirmed by the electron microscopic appearances of the canaliculi, which during cholestasis quickly lose their microvilli and become dilated. On routine light microscopy yellow-brown 'bile plugs' may be seen within them. The canalicular membrane may become more permeable, so allowing water to pass out until the bile becomes too

20    *Chapter 2*

concentrated and precipitates as solid bile plugs.

The histological appearances of extrahepatic cholestasis include swelling and oedema of the portal tracts and their infiltration by polymorphonuclear leucocytes, proliferation of small bile ductules in the tracts, and bilirubin-stained areas of liver cell necrosis (bile lakes) within the lobules. But it can still be difficult to distinguish histologically extrahepatic from intrahepatic cholestasis.

Clincally, intrahepatic and extrahepatic cholestasis both similarly cause jaundice, itching, and raised levels of conjugated bilirubin, alkaline phosphatase and bile acids in blood. If cholestasis is longstanding cholesterol levels also rise.

## CHOLESTEROL

Cholesterol is an essential component of cell membranes and the precursor of bile acids and steroid hormones. Some is derived from the diet, but the major portion is synthesised chiefly in the cells of the intestinal mucosa and liver. After esterification with fatty acids by the enzyme lecithin cholesterol acyl transferase (LCAT), it is carried in the blood in particles of protein and phospholipid (lipoproteins).

In prolonged cholestasis, the level of cholesterol in blood rises, but most is then not esterified. This may be due to a defect in LCAT. In addition, reflux of phospholipids from the liver keeps more cholesterol in the blood.

In extreme cases cholesterol is deposited in the skin and tendons as xanthomata (*see* chapter 1).

## Bile acids

### HEPATIC METABOLISM

The two *primary* bile acids, the trihydroxy cholic and dihydroxy chenodeoxycholic (chenic) acids, are synthesised at the rate of 200–600 mg daily by the liver from cholesterol (Figure 2.5). Their rate of synthesis is controlled by the amount of bile acids returning from the intestine to the liver in portal venous blood. Oral administration of bile acids reduces their hepatic synthesis, while reducing the amount returning from the intestine increases it, although only to a maximum of about 1 g daily.

Bile acids reduce synthesis by inhibiting the activity of the enzyme 7 $\alpha$-hydroxylase, which is rate limiting in the conversion of cholesterol to bile acids. Like bilirubin, bile acids are conjugated in liver cells, but with glycine or taurine, normally in a ratio of 2:1, glycine : taurine (Figure 2.5). The conjugated acids are then secreted into bile carrying water with them (bile acid dependent bile flow; see above).

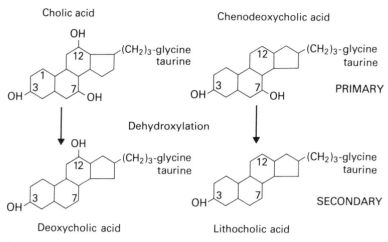

**Figure 2.5** Primary and secondary bile acids.

## ENTEROHEPATIC CIRCULATION

In the upper small intestine conjugated bile acids are not absorbed much until they reach the terminal ileum, from where they return unchanged to the liver in portal venous blood and are re-excreted into bile. This is an enterohepatic circulation (Figure 2.6), similar to that of urobilinogen. Conjugation prevents absorption in the jejunum, for unconjugated bile acids are rapidly absorbed. If this were not so, the concentration of bile acids within the lumen of the small intestine would be too low to aid in digestion (see p. 24).

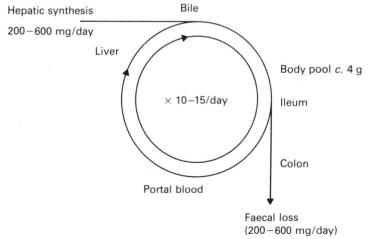

**Fig. 2.6** Enterohepatic circulation of bile acids.

22                                    *Chapter 2*

During meals bile acids circulate in this way 6–8 times between intestine and liver. The total bile acids in the body, namely the bile acid pool, is almost 4 g, and only 1% of this is lost into the faeces during one circulation, so about 15% of the pool is lost each day and has to be replaced by bile acids newly synthesised in the liver.

Less than 5% of conjugated bile acids in the small intestine escape on through the ileocæcal valve into the colon, where cholic and chenodeoxycholic acids are deconjugated and dehydroxylated to the *secondary* bile acids, deoxycholic (dihydroxy) and lithocholic (monohydroxy) acids respectively.

Deoxycholic acid is reabsorbed from the colon, but most of the lithocholic acid is excreted into faeces. Deoxycholic acid in portal venous blood is removed by the liver and like the primary bile acids is conjugated with glycine and taurine, excreted into bile and then also undergoes an enterohepatic circulation.

So six glycine or taurine conjugated bile acids are continuously undergoing this circulation (Figure 2.5). There are also small quantities of other bile acids, such as lithocholic and ursodeoxycholic acids.

## MICELLES

The main function of bile acids is to act as detergents in bile and the small intestine. They do this by spontaneously forming tiny submicroscopic aggregates or micelles, which are about 10 nm in diameter and contain about ten molecules of bile acid (Figure 2.7). But they do this only if their concentration exceeds about 1.0 mM, which is called the *critical micellar concentration*. Unconjugated bile acids do this almost as well as their conjugates, so conjugation is chiefly a mechanism to slow their absorption from the jejunum, rather than improve their physiochemical micellar properties.

In bile, the micelles also contain inside them the phospholipid lecithin, and are then called *mixed micelles*. They have a lower critical micellar concentration and can carry more insoluble lipid than simple bile acid micelles. The shape of a micelle is something like a tin of asparagus, the bile acids lining up on the outside with their water soluble hydroxyl and carboxyl groups facing outwards into the water and their lipid soluble groups inwards, forming an inner lipophilic environment.

The bile acid molecule is termed *amphipathic* (liking both water and lipid) and this makes them good detergents, which means they can dissolve lipids in water.

This dissolution occurs as lipid soluble molecules enter the micelles where they are kept in a lipid environment away from the surrounding water. In bile, cholesterol is the chief lipid that is carried in this way; otherwise

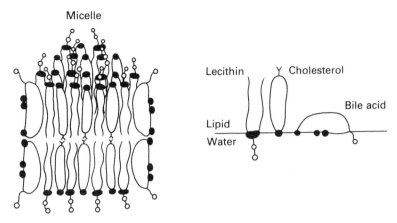

**Fig. 2.7** Orientation of cholesterol, lecithin and bile acid at a lipid:water interface, and their formation into a micelle.

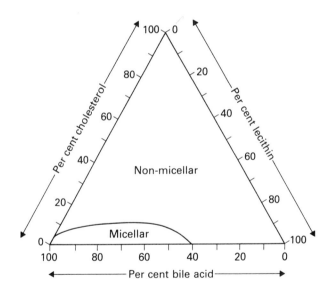

**Fig. 2.8** Triangular coordinates of relative concentrations of cholesterol, lecithin and bile acid that form micelles.

it would precipitate.

Only a small amount of cholesterol can be carried by a micelle of bile acids and lecithin. The relative proportions of bile acids and lecithin needed to keep a given amount of cholesterol in solution can be shown on a

24                                    *Chapter 2*

triangular diagram (Figure 2.8), with the coordinates of cholesterol, bile acid and lecithin concentrations. Outside a small area in the diagram cholesterol is not fully dissolved and precipitates.

In the intestine micelles carry the products of fat digestion, namely fatty acids and monoglycerides, and take them to the intestinal wall where they are absorbed into the mucosa. The bile acids remain in the lumen, however, and continue to solubilise lipids, when they reach the ileum they are finally absorbed themselves and pass back to the liver in enterohepatic circulation.

## BILE ACIDS AND CHOLESTASIS

During cholestasis bile acids, like bilirubin, cannot be fully excreted into bile, and so accumulate in blood and tissues, even though their hepatic synthesis is suppressed. It has been thought that bile acids in the skin cause the itching of liver disease, but this is unlikely.

Raised amounts of bile acids pass into urine, and, being detergents, they lower its surface tension and cause it to froth.

## BILE ACIDS AND MALABSORPTION

A shortage of bile acids in the intestinal lumen occurs in liver disease, especially if there is cholestasis. If their concentration falls below the critical micellar concentration fat absorption is impaired, causing steatorrhoea and diarrhoea, and malabsorption of fat soluble vitamins.

Steatorrhoea is particularly prominent in patients with primary biliary cirrhosis (*see* chapter 10) and may be an early feature of this disease. It is treated with a low fat diet and oral codeine phosphate (30–180 mg daily in divided doses).

### Protein synthesis

### ALBUMIN

Serum albumin is made entirely in liver cells. The normal level is 38–48 g/litre, and the total pool about 300 g, much being in lymph and interstitial fluid. The protein has a half-life time of 20 days. It contributes more than other plasma proteins to the osmotic pressure of blood.

In chronic liver disease the capacity of the liver to synthesise albumin fails, and also albumin becomes abnormally distributed between vascular and extravascular spaces. Hence serum albumin levels fall.

Globulins are made in lymphocytes throughout the body, and not in hepatocytes, and so their levels do not fall in liver disease.

## COAGULATION FACTORS

The liver is central in the coagulation of blood. Many of the coagulation factors, namely I (fibrinogen), II (prothrombin), V, VII, IX and X are synthesised solely in liver cells, as are inhibitors of clotting. Factors II, V, VII and IX are called *prothrombin complex factors*. VIII is made in reticuloendothelial cells in the liver and elsewhere, and not in hepatocytes.

Severe acute or chronic liver cell failure alters coagulation in several ways.

**1.** There is hepatic protein synthesis, including coagulation factors, and this causes impaired clotting of blood, which is seen as easy skin bruising, purpura, and gastrointestinal and nasal bleeding.

**2.** In severe liver disease intravascular coagulation also occurs, particularly in acute hepatic necrosis, and fibrinolysis may also be abnormally active.

**3.** The reticuloendothelial cells of the liver normally remove the products of clotting, such a fibrin, from blood and this may fail.

**4.** Platelets can be reduced in number and activity due to bone marrow failure, hypersplenism and consumption during intravascular coagulation.

**5.** The lipid soluble vitamin K is needed for the synthesis of the prothrombin complex factors in liver cells (Figure 2.9), and so another reason for abnormal clotting in liver disease is a deficiency of this vitamin due to its malabsorption from the bowel (*see* p. 24).

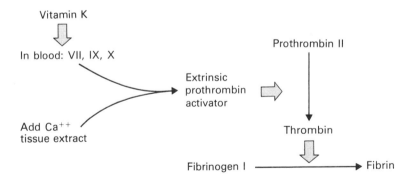

**Fig. 2.9** Coagulation cascade and site of action of vitamin K.

Not surprisingly, therefore, severe coagulation problems in liver disease are complex and difficult to treat. Fresh frozen plasma or concentrates of clotting factors may be given, but their effect is only temporary.

# 26 *Chapter 2*

## Drug metabolism

The metabolism of the many drugs that are detoxified and excreted by the liver is impaired in liver disease, though these changes are seldom of clinical importance. The causes are manifold, and include reduction of effective liver blood-flow, failure of conjugation and metabolism in the liver cells, failure of excretion and cholestasis, altered binding of drugs to plasma proteins, and changed non-hepatic end-organ sensitivity.

Thus sedative drugs are likely to precipitate encephalopathy in liver failure, partly due to increased cerebral sensitivity. Opiates are particularly dangerous, but no sedative is completely safe.

## Endocrine change

### SEX HORMONES

The clinical features of altered balance of sex hormones in liver disease namely amenorrhoea, gynaecomastia, loss of body hair, impotence and testicular atrophy (and perhaps spider naevi and palmar erythema) were thought to be due to poor removal of hormones by the abnormal liver. However, the secretion rates of hormones are often normal and direct toxicity of alcohol on the gonads may be more important.

### INSULIN

Diabetes is frequent in cirrhosis, due not to impaired hepatic metabolism, but to an ill-understood impairment of the peripheral uptake of glucose. Insulin is not usually needed for treatment; oral hypoglycaemic drugs suffice.

In haemochromatosis the iron laid down in the pancreas frequently causes diabetes.

Hypoglycaemia occasionally occurs in fulminant liver failure, particularly in fatty liver of pregnancy (*see* chapter 14), presumably because the severely damaged liver cannot maintain glycogen breakdown, gluconeogenesis, and thus blood glucose levels. It is also sometimes seen after an alcoholic binge.

### ENCEPHALOPATHY

The increasing drowsiness, flapping tremor, fetor, stupor, and eventually coma of encephalopathy (*see* chapter 1) are ominous signs of severe and often irreversible, acute (due to severe hepatitis), or chronic (from advanced cirrhosis) liver failure. Histological changes in the brain *post mortem*

*Pathophysiology and Treatment of Complications* 27

are slight, although cerebral oedema, raised intracranial pressure and coning of the temporal lobes through the tentorium may occur terminally. The electroencephalogram shows slowing, and eventually flattening, of the cerebral electrical waves, but this is not specific for hepatic encephalopathy.

Encephalopathy is caused by a combination of liver cell failure and shunting of blood both straight *through* the liver avoiding the sinusoids and functioning liver cells (intrahepatic shunts), and *around* the liver via extrahepatic blood vessels (extrahepatic shunts). The biochemical changes are due to failure of the liver to remove, or less likely, add something to the blood perfusing the brain.

There are many noxious substances present in high concentration in the blood of patients with encephalopathy, such as:

Amino acids
Amines (false neurotransmitters)
Short-chain fatty acids
Ammonium
Acidosis
Low cerebral blood flow

All can be shown experimentally to depress cerebral function, and their effects may, therefore, combine to produce the encephalopathy.

Some causes that precipitate encephalopathy are:

Constipation
Infections
Over-use of diuretics
Hypokalaemia
Gastrointestinal haemorrhage
Sedative drugs
Portal-caval shunts
Therapeutic paracentesis

Some of the amines and amino acids might act as false neurotransmitters, that is, their structure is similar enough to true neurotransmitters to combine with their receptors in the brain and block their action.

## Treatment

Treatment of encephalopathy will involve:

Treatment of precipitating cause
Lactulose 30–200 ml daily

28 *Chapter 2*

Enemata
Low protein diet
Oral neomycin, 4 g daily
Dexamethasone

Any possible precipitating cause should be considered and vigorously treated. Since the aetiology is unknown, there is no specific treatment. However, treatment may involve:

**1.** The bowels being kept empty of blood and faeces, preferably with the oral laxative lactulose (30–200 ml of 67 g/100 ml elixir daily). If necessary this can be given through a nasogastric tube if the patient is comatose. This is beneficial chiefly by emptying the bowel. Being an osmotic laxative, it passes unabsorbed down the intestine to the colon where bacteria degrade it. In addition, its bacterial metabolism makes the colonic pH more acid, and this inhibits the growth of bacteria that release toxic amines and amino acids, and also reduces the absorption of ammonium into the blood.

Rectal washouts and enemata may be needed, but blood is a good laxative!

**2.** A low protein diet (40 g daily) will reduce the absorption of nitrogenous products from the intestine.

**3.** The poorly absorbed antibiotic neomycin is given orally (1g qds) since this reduces the intestinal bacterial flora. Prolonged administration, however, can cause irreversible nerve deafness.

**4.** Cerebral oedema occurs when there is coma in terminal acute liver failure, and treatment with the steroid dexamethasone (2–4 mg tds) may improve this.

## THE KIDNEY AND THE LIVER

The kidney and the liver may be linked in several pathological ways, all loosely called *hepatorenal syndromes*.

### Hepatorenal syndromes

### SINGLE AETIOLOGY

Leptospirosis (*see* chapter 6) and certain poisons, such as chloroform, damage the cells of both organs. Polycystic disease may develop in both organs.

# Pathophysiology and Treatment of Complications

## SURGERY AND JAUNDICE

In jaundiced patients there is an increased susceptibility to acute renal failure after surgical operations, possibly due to the toxic effects of both conjugated bilirubin and bile acids on the renal tubules. Mannitol (100 ml of 10% solution) is given intravenously during surgery on jaundiced patients to protect the kidney.

## INTRAVASCULAR COAGULATION

In severe acute liver failure widespread intravascular coagulation damages both kidney and liver.

## TRUE HEPATORENAL SYNDROME

In patients with cirrhosis, a slowly increasing oliguria and deterioration of renal function may occur. This is the true hepatorenal syndrome.

It is usually prerenal failure, that is without proteinuria, and with normal histological appearances on renal biopsy. There is intense sodium absorption from the tubular fluid and less than 20 mmol sodium is excreted daily, but the urine remains concentrated with relatively high osmolality.

The serum creatinine rises, and although the plasma urea also rises, its level is lower than expected because its synthesis from ammonium in liver cells is reduced. Paradoxically, in plasma there is hyponatraemia, even though there is an overall excess of intracellular sodium in the body. It can be precipitated by the use of diuretics, by infections and by hypotension.

The cause of this syndrome is not clear, but there is a reduced blood flow through the renal cortex, and this may be due to increased circulating levels of bacterial endotoxins, amines or kinins absorbed from the intestine and not detoxified by the sick liver.

Even though it is a prerenal failure, in advanced liver disease it is often irreversible and precedes death.

### Treatment

Infections and hypovolaemia must be treated. Correcting hyponatraemia with saline is fruitless and dangerous. Diuretic therapy should be reduced. Intravenous infusions of human salt-poor albumin have been tried. Dialysis is not effective. The prognosis of the established syndrome is poor.

## RENAL TUBULAR NECROSIS

Occasionally intrinsic damage to the kidney occurs in cirrhosis or severe hepatitis with the picture of renal tubular necrosis. Hypotension from gastrointestinal haemorrhage can be the cause. Urine sodium is more than 20 mmol daily, and the urine becomes isomolar with plasma, since it cannot be concentrated by the kidney. It is usually reversible.

## PORTAL HYPERTENSION

### Haemodynamics

The liver receives about 1500 ml blood per minute (20 ml/kg body weight) or a third of the cardiac output. One third, i.e. 500 ml, is carried in the hepatic artery, which is one of the three major branches of the coeliac axis, and two thirds in the portal vein. Normally all the blood draining the intestinal tract, other than the oesophagus and rectum, passes through the liver

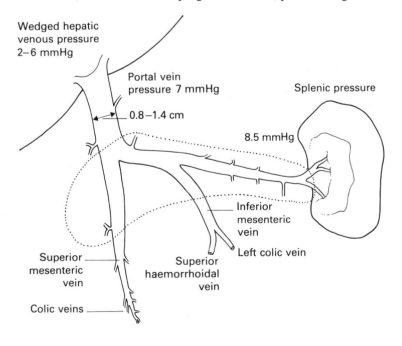

**Fig. 2.10**   Anatomy and pressures of the portal venous system.

in the portal venous system (Figure 2.10). The arterial and venous blood probably fully mix and their different pressures equalise in the portal tracts so that mixed blood perfuses across the lobule in the sinusoids (*see* below).

The pressure in the portal vein is only about 8–12 mm Hg and slightly higher in its tributaries. There is little resistance to flow in the liver so that the pressure in the hepatic veins draining the liver is about 5 mmHg, this being enough to carry the blood into the inferior vena cava and the right atrium.

Any increase of resistance to the flow leads to *portal hypertension*, the pressure in the portal vein then rising to as high as 40 mmHg. Portal hypertension is usually divided into presinusoidal and postsinusoidal types, judged by hepatic vein catheter pressure measurements (*see* chapter 3).

### Presinusoidal portal hypertension

The obstruction to flow lies before the blood reaches the hepatic sinusoid (Figure 2.11). Liver cell function is well preserved, and pressure in the sinusoids is normal.

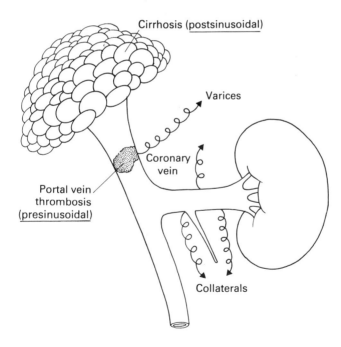

**Fig. 2.11**  Presinusoidal (portal vein thrombosis) and postsinusoidal (cirrhosis) portal hypertension.

32 *Chapter 2*

It is uncommon, but it can be due to extrahepatic or intrahepatic causes (Table 2.2). Thus thrombosis of the portal vein is an example of the former, causing so-called left-sided portal hypertension.

**Table 2.2** Causes of portal hypertension.

|  | Presinusoidal | Postsinusoidal |
| --- | --- | --- |
| Extrahepatic | Thrombosis<br>Sepsis<br>Tumours<br>Blood dyscrasias<br>Pancreatitis<br>Pregnancy<br><br>Increased splenic flow<br>'Primary'<br>Reticuloses<br>Fistulae | Budd-Chiari syndrome<br>Polycythaemia<br>Contraceptive pill<br>Tumours<br>Congenital webs |
| Intrahepatic | Portal tract damage<br>Schistosomiasis<br>Sarcoidosis<br>Congenital hepatic fibrosis<br>Reticulosis | Cirrhosis<br>Veno-occulusive disease |

Schistosomiasis (*see* chapter 6) is a common cause of portal hypertension in tropical countries, and leads to an intrahepatic, presinusoidal block due to fibrosis in the portal tracts.

Sometimes splenomegaly alone may increase flow into the portal system enough to cause hypertension without any pathological obstruction in the liver. Lymphomata or storage diseases are cause of this, as is the strange splenomegaly in tropical areas where malaria is endemic.

### Postsinusoidal portal hypertension

Postsinusoidal portal hypertension (see Figure 2.11) is much more common in the UK than presinusoidal, but is usually a mixture of postsinusoidal and presinusoidal obstruction. Cirrhosis is the major cause in all countries of

# Pathophysiology and Treatment of Complications

the world, the regeneration nodules probably compressing intrahepatic hepatic veins. Pressure in the hepatic sinusoids is raised.

A more dramatic postsinusoidal obstruction is produced when the major hepatic veins are blocked by a tumour or thrombosis. This is called the Budd-Chiari syndrome (*see* chapter 12).

Liver function is usually much worse in postsinusoidal than presinusoidal portal hypertension.

## VARICES

In both presinusoidal and postsinusoidal hypertension, as the pressure rises in the portal venous system, collateral veins open up in an attempt to shunt portal blood directly into the systemic venous circulation, rather than through the obstructed liver or portal vein. These collaterals eventually become numerous, large, and tortuous, feeding backwards through the mesentery to the renal veins and inferior vena cava, and up into the chest around the

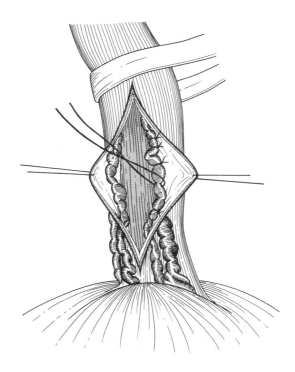

**Fig. 2.12** Submucosal oesophageal veins and deep para-oesophageal veins.

34 *Chapter 2*

oesophagus to join the azygous venous system (Figure 2.12). They are occasionally so effective that the portal pressure returns to normal.

Although most of the collateral vessels do little harm apart from shunting intestinal blood into the systemic circulation (*see* encephalopathy, p. 26), those running in the submucosa of the oesophagus and stomach form protruding varices that are liable to rupture and bleed. Larger varices probably bleed more than smaller ones, but it is uncertain why they suddenly start to bleed.

## GASTROINTESTINAL HAEMORRHAGE

Bleeding from the oesophagus and stomach is common in advanced liver disease, due to rupture of the submucosal varices plus poor clotting of the blood. There is also an increased incidence of acute erosions of the gastric mucosa, and of peptic ulcers. Alcoholics are particularly liable to develop erosions and ulcers. Haematemesis and melaena are therefore common, but if the bleeding is slow only melaena and anaemia may occur.

However, in the UK only 5% of all patients admitted to hospital for gastrointestinal haemorrhage are bleeding from varices.

### Diagnosis

A history of alcoholism, liver disease or previous haemorrhage will suggest that it is varices, rather than an ulcer, that are bleeding. The presence of signs of encephalopathy (flap, stupor), fluid retention (ascites, oedema), portal hypertension (palpable spleen), and abnormal clotting may suggest liver disease, and also therefore, the possibility of variceal bleeding. A more sure diagnosis should always be obtained with a barium swallow X-ray or, preferably, gastroscopy (*see* chapter 3).

### Treatment

Treatment is initially similar to that for patients without liver disease, but the underlying health of liver patients is poor. Bleeding from varices is particularly difficult to control.

Treatment of bleeding varices may include:

Transfusion, clotting factors vitamin K; $H^2$-antagonist
Barium swallow/gastroscopy
Intravenous vasopressin (20–40 units/hour)
Emergency endoscopic sclerosis
Sengstaken balloon tube
Emergency surgery

*Pathophysiology and Treatment of Complications* 35

## TRANSFUSION

Blood volume is best restored with fresh blood as the patient with cirrhosis is likely to be deficient in the clotting factors. Central venous catheter measurements are useful in assessing right atrial pressure and transfusion requirements.

## CLOTTING FACTORS

With clotting abnormalities, if the prothrombin time is prolonged, 10 mg of vitamin K is administered intramuscularly or intravenously once on two successive days. Fresh plasma or clotting factor concentrates can be given.

## FLUIDS

Dextrose rather than saline is given between transfusions as many patients with liver disease already have an excess of sodium in their cells.

## NASOGASTRIC TUBE

It is best not to pass a nasogastric tube unless the patient is unconscious and liable to inhale vomited blood. It may cause oesophagitis, rupture varices, or chest infections, and is unpleasant for the patient.

### Definitive treatment

## DRUG THERAPY

Bleeding peptic ulcers are treated, probably ineffectually, with intravenous and then oral cimetidine 1 g or ranitidine 300 mg daily in divided doses, or by surgery if bleeding cannot be stopped.

Acute gastric erosions are effectively treated with cimetidine 1 g daily or ranitidine in divided doses; surgery is not advisable. Oral antacids may help.

Bleeding gastric or oesophageal varices are vigorously treated, since any intestinal bleeding increases encephalopathy and probably reduces liver blood flow and function.

## VASOPRESSIN ADMINISTRATION

Vasopressin is administered at a dose of 0.4–0.8 units/kg body weight/hour, or about 0.4–0.8 units/minute (24–48 units/hour) in adults, by continuous intravenous infusion in dextrose for 24–48 hours. Single bolus injections

36 *Chapter 2*

of 20 units were once used, but are less effective.

Vasopressin constricts mesenteric and other arterioles, and reduces blood flow through the liver and the portal pressure, and therefore the pressure in the varices. It may therefore reduce bleeding from varices, gastric erosions and peptic ulcers. It has been given by direct infusion through an arterial catheter into the superior mesenteric artery, but this technique is difficult, and complications such as intestinal necrosis occur. Peripheral intravenous infusions are as effective and safer. Ideally the right atrial pressure should be monitored as venoconstriction can cause right sided cardiac failure. Confusion, angina and intestinal colic can occur also during treatment, but rapidly improve if the dose is reduced.

### SENGSTAKEN TUBE

If vasopressin fails, a four-lumen *Sengstaken tube* is placed in the stomach and oesophagus (Figure 2.13), but only after endoscopy has confirmed that the source of the bleeding is varices. The patient swallows the lubricated tube, and the gastric balloon is inflated with air or gastrografin to about 500 ml, and the oesophageal balloon to a pressure of 30–45 mmHg monitored with a manometer. Blood and stomach contents are aspired via the third, gastric lumen, and saliva from the upper oesophagus above the oesophageal balloon through the fourth lumen.

The tube is taped to the patient's cheek. Ideally a nurse is present constantly in case the tube should slip out of place and obstruct the airway. A plain abdominal X-ray will confirm the correct positioning of the tube. The patient will need to have careful sedation as this procedure is most unpleasant.

The apparatus presumably compresses the varices and aids clotting, but it may also divert blood away from the oesophageal submucosal veins into the azygous veins. It should be deflated after 24 hours, and then if bleeding restarts injection and surgery considered.

### INJECTION OF VARICES

Somewhat similar to the injection of haemorrhoids in the rectum, oesophageal varices can be injected at the bottom of the oesophagus with a long needle (Figure 2.14). This is not suitable for gastric varices. It may be carried out using a rigid metal oesophagoscope with the patient under general anaesthesia or by using a flexible, fibreoptic endoscope while the patient is given intravenous sedation. If necessary, a Sengstaken tube can be inserted after the procedure.

Injection is most effective in preventing rebleeding when varices have

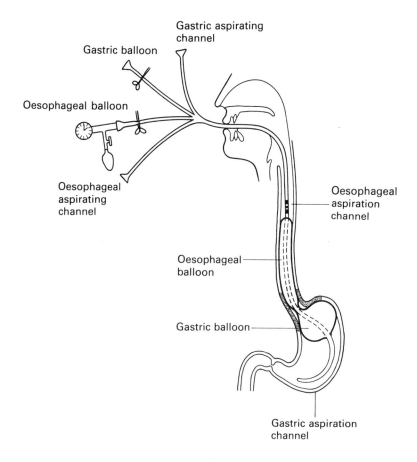

**Fig. 2.13** Four-lumen Sengstaken tube in place to compress bleeding varices.

temporarily stopped bleeding; it is more difficult when there is blood in the oesophagus. Ethanolamine oleate in oil or sodium tetradecyl sulphate is used. It reduces bleeding by fibrosing the submucosa and veins. Repeated injections at intervals are needed to obliterate them. Occasionally strictures develop after injections.

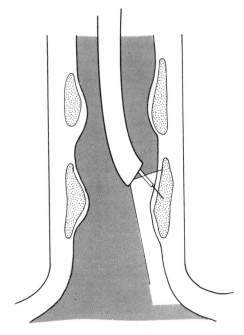

**Fig. 2.14**  Injection of lower oesophageal varices via a fibreoptic endoscope.

## SURGERY

Oesophageal varices may be approached directly through the chest or abdomen or indirectly decompressed by one of several portal decompression procedures or shunts. Results are poor in sick patients with cirrhosis and uncontrolled bleeding, i.e., when done as an *emergency* procedure, but better in patients whose bleeding has stopped, i.e., as an *elective* procedure.

Emergency surgery may include: transection of the oesophagus; oversewing of varices via a thoracotomy; devascularisation of the stomach; or transection of the abdominal oesophagus, using a stapling gun or a Boerema Button, through the abdomen.

The portal vein may be directly anastomosed to the inferior vena cava using the end-to-side (Figure 2.15) or side-to-side (Figure 2.16) portal caval shunt. In one method the end of the transected portal vein is connected to the side of the cava, and in the other the sides are joined preserving portal flow into the liver. The merits of the two are debated, but the former is technically easier.

Other operations include the spleno-renal shunt (splenic vein to left renal vein), which includes splenectomy; the mesenteric caval shunt, often using

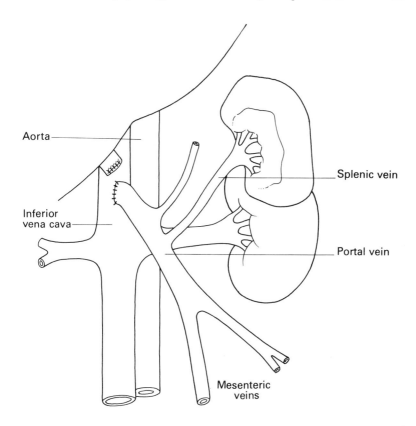

**Figure 2.15** End-to-side portal caval shunt.

a prosthetic graft between the inferior vena cava and superior mesenteric vein; and, more recently, the distal splenorenal (Warren) shunt, in which the spleen is preserved, and the splenic vein divided and the distal (splenic) end used to drain the gastric and oesophageal blood down into the left renal vein (Figure 2.17).

## General treatment

The bowels are kept open with the laxative lactulose (30–200 ml of the elixir — 67 g/100 ml), a low protein diet (40 g daily) and neomycin given to reduce encephalopathy (*see previously*).

The frequent chest infections and any other infections are vigorously treated with antibiotics and fluid retention reduced with diuretics (*see later*).

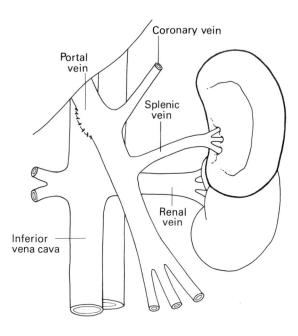

**Fig. 2.16**   Side-to-side portal caval shunt.

Vitamins include B complex (as Parentrovite), C and folic acid are needed in the alcoholic patient.

*Beware* sedation with drugs that increase encephalopathy, although they may be needed for the restless patient and when a Sengstaken tube is in place, diazepam or chlormethiazole are the safest drugs, but are still dangerous.

## SPLENOMEGALY

A large spleen is not uncommon in patients with liver disease, and often becomes palpable if there is portal hypertension. However, the size of the spleen is poorly correlated with the degree of portal hypertension, the size of oesophageal varices or their chance of bleeding. Splenomegaly is also no indication of liver function. Patients can die from liver cell failure due to cirrhosis without a palpable spleen, while in schistosomiasis a large spleen usually coexists with good liver function.

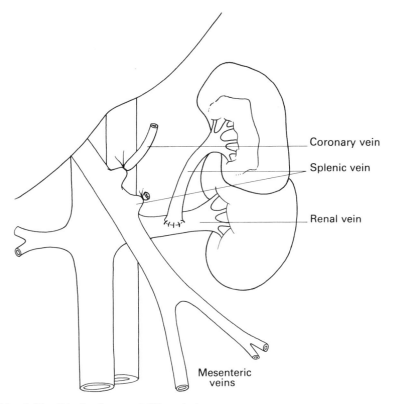

**Fig. 2.17** Distal splenorenal (Warren) shunt.

## Diagnosis

### PAIN

A dragging left-sided discomfort or sometimes pain can be caused by a large spleen.

### PORTAL HYPERTENSION

The spleen does *not* enlarge in response to the increased portal pressure, and indeed the increased flow through it contributes to portal pressure. In tropical splenomegaly, and occasionally with splenomegaly due to lymphoma, presinusoidal portal hypertension with varices develops without any liver disease, and then is solely due to increased blood flow into a normal venous system.

42 *Chapter 2*

## PANCYTOPENIA

The large spleen causes blood to pool in its sinusoids, and there excessive destruction of red and white blood cells and platelets occurs, namely *hypersplenism*. In addition the total plasma volume may be increased by up to 50%, and this further reduces the concentrations of the formed elements in the blood. Severely depressed levels, however, are unusual. The leucopenia may contribute to the increased susceptibility of patients with liver disease to infections.

## Aetiology

One hypothesis for the aetiology of splenomegaly is that it is due to bacterial and viral antigens absorbed from the gut bypassing the normal efficient filtering action of the liver, through the collateral vessels, and reaching the systemic circulation. The lymphoid tissue of the spleen therefore hypertrophies in response to these circulating antigens, which it helps to clear from the blood. This situation is illustrated by the increased uptake of colloidal particles by the spleen when a liver scan (*see* chapter 3) is performed in patients with cirrhosis.

## Treatment

Splenectomy as a primary operation is seldom indicated in liver disease, unless it is a mandatory part of a shunt operation, such as a splenorenal shunt. It can be considered if splenic pain is pronounced, if there is severe thrombocytopenia, or if there is prehepatic presinusoidal portal hypertension. The removal of a large spleen, however, is hazardous, does not cure hepatic portal hypertension, and may be followed by dangerous thrombocythaemia and by septicaemia.

## ELECTROLYTE AND WATER BALANCE

### Ascites and oedema

Ascites and oedema are common features, and sometimes the presenting symptoms, of chronic liver disease. Their pathophysiology is complex, but includes the retention and redistribution of salt and water.

The aetiology of hepatic oedema involves:

*Pathophysiology and Treatment of Complications* 43

Renal sodium retention (*hyperaldosteronism*)
Low serum albumin
Portal hypertension
Inappropriate antidiuretic hormone
Third factor reduction

## EFFECTS ON BODY

### Salt and water retention

The total content of sodium in the body may be increased by up to 100% in patients with cirrhosis, even though at the same time they may be excreting less than 10 mmol of sodium daily in the urine (normal 30–120 mmol). There is therefore intense, but inappropriate, retention of sodium due to reabsorption from the glomerular filtrate. Why?

One reason is inappropriately high blood concentration of aldosterone, or *secondary hyperaldosteronism*, which also occurs in cardiac failure. This causes increased renal sodium reabsorption and potassium excretion. The reason for hyperaldosteronism, however, is unknown.

Secondly, there may be reduced production of the so-called 'third factor', which is thought to promote renal sodium excretion.

Thirdly, there is reduced blood flow through the renal cortex, and therefore reduced supply to the glomeruli and reduced glomerular filtration of urine. This causes a decreased load of sodium to, and increased reabsorption of sodium from, the proximal tubules. The maldistribution of renal blood may be due to increased blood levels of vasoactive compounds that are usually removed by the liver.

Finally, blood levels of antidiuretic hormone are elevated and will increase water reabsorption in the distal tubule.

### Fluid redistribution

A low serum albumin level is almost invariable in patients with ascites and oedema from liver disease (*see later*). The plasma osmotic pressure is therefore low and allows water to leave the circulation into the tissue. This contributes to the reduced plasma volume in patients with severe liver disease.

In liver disease excess tissue fluid accumulates in the abdomen as ascites because there is increased hydrostatic pressure in the abdominal venules due to portal hypertension. Secondly, lymphatic drainage through the liver is impaired in cirrhosis, and thirdly the blockage of the hepatic venous drainage by regeneration nodules also increases the formation of lymph in the liver, and this exudes into the peritoneal cavity.

44 *Chapter 2*

The ascitic fluid in cirrhosis is often therefore a transudate with a low protein concentration, but if it contains lymph, it is sometimes a protein rich exudate with albumin concentrations greater than 40 g/litre. Still higher protein concentrations are found when the ascites is infected, and sometimes when a malignant hepatoma develops. In general, however, it is not helpful to measure ascitic protein levels.

Infection of the ascitic fluid by tubercle bacilli and *Streptococcus pneumoniae* can occur in liver disease.

### TREATMENT

A few millilitres of ascitic fluid should be removed for analysis for malignant and pus cells, and for microbiological culture.

Removal of large quantities of ascitic fluid, that is *therapeutic paracentesis*, is dangerous and ineffective, and therefore rarely indicated. It is dangerous because the sudden removal of fluid and subsequent rapid refilling of the peritoneal cavity reduces plasma volume and liver blood flow and may increase liver cell failure, because precious albumin in the fluid is removed, and because infection is easily introduced. It is ineffective because the ascites rapidly reaccumulates in a few days.

Treatment is directed at reversing the sodium and fluid retention and involves:

> Stopping table salt intake
> Administering diuretics
> Performing a peritoneo-venous shunt

#### Low salt diet

A low salt diet is much used, but is not usually necessary since modern diuretics are so powerful. It is worth stopping the patient adding salt to food at the table, but a rigid diet may be unpalatable.

#### Diuretics

A diuresis can be obtained with increasing doses of spironolactone, which is an aldosterone antagonist, and therefore a logical diuretic to use in liver disease. The patient is started on 50–100 mg once daily, increasing the dose every few days; patients resistant to treatment may need 150–1000 mg once daily. A slow, controlled diuresis can be obtained, and without risk of potassium depletion.

Frusemide 40–120 mg daily can be added if the response is poor. This is beneficial by reducing the more proximal reabsorption of sodium. This may otherwise be so intense that there is insufficient sodium reaching the distal tubule for spironolactone to cause sodium loss. Frusemide is not given as the first line of treatment, however, as it would be in a patient with heart failure. There is a greater risk of potassium depletion, and a dangerously large and sudden diuresis can occur in liver disease. Too rapid diuresis can increase liver failure by reducing plasma volume.

If there is ascites the patient is put to bed, since this aids the initiation of the diuresis, and is weighed daily. A weight, and therefore fluid, loss of 0.5 kg daily is aimed for, but seldom exactly achieved. The patient with oedema alone can usually be treated as an out-patient.

Occasionally patients are resistant even to spironolactone plus frusemide. They usually have poor liver function, and there is hyponatraemia and a low plasma volume, i.e. the hepatorenal syndrome (*see* p. 28). This syndrome is seldom reversible.

Increasing the dose of diuretics only reduces plasma volume more and causes more uraemia.

### *Peritoneo-venous shunt*

Recently, removal of the ascitic fluid through a peritoneal catheter and simply reinfusing it into a peripheral vein (LeVeen peritoneo-venous shunt) has been tried with some success. Surprisingly the procedure is often followed by a diuresis.

## VITAMIN DEFICIENCIES

### Water soluble vitamins

### VITAMIN B

In the alcoholic patient, with or without liver disease, dietary vitamin $B_1$ (thiamine) deficiency may occur.

Beri-beri is rare in this country, but Wernicke's encephalopathy, which is also due to thiamine deficiency, occurs sometimes and is easily missed. It presents as confusion and stupor, with nystagmus, small pupils, cranial nerve palsies and ataxia, but sometimes without any of these classical physical signs. Treatment is **urgent** as the condition becomes irreversible.

Riboflavin and nicotinamide ($B_2$) deficiency may also occur, but recent work suggests that pyridoxine ($B_6$) deficiency may be more common. Treatment is with the B complex vitamins intravenously or intramuscularly as Parentrovite (containing thiamine, riboflavin, pyridoxine, nicotinamide and ascorbic acid) twice, with later oral supplements.

46 *Chapter 2*

## VITAMIN C AND FOLIC ACID

Vitamin C and folic acid deficiencies are common, and both vitamins should be given to patients with alcoholic liver disease, 100 mg vitamin C and 10 mg folic acid orally per day.

### Fat soluble vitamins

Fat soluble vitamins require micellar concentrations of bile acids in the intestine for their absorption, and are therefore poorly absorbed in chronic cholestasis.

## VITAMIN A

Vitamin A deficiency is uncommon, but can cause night blindness. Treatment is with 100 000 units intramuscularly, monthly.

## VITAMIN D

Vitamin D deficiency is more common. Vitamin D is eaten as cholecalciferol (vitamin $D_3$) or calciferol (ergocalciferol, $D_2$), or as precursors that are converted to $D_3$ in the skin on exposure to sunlight. In the liver, $D_3$ is hydroxylated by a microsomal enzyme to 25-hydroxyvitamin D (25 (OH) $D_3$), which is partly excreted in bile and reabsorbed, thus undergoing an enterohepatic circulation. It is then further hydroxylated in the kidney to 1,25 dihydroxyvitamin $D_3$ (1,25(OH)$_2D_3$), which is the active hormone.

In chronic cholestasis and in alcoholism a combination of factors may produce vitamin D deficiency. The diet may be inadequate in $D_3$, exposure to sun is reduced, especially as many cholestatic patients find their itching is worse in the sunlight, hepatic hydroxylation may be impaired, and finally the enterohepatic circulation of 25 (OH) $D_3$ may be impaired because of intestinal bile acid deficiency and malabsorption.

Vitamin D deficiency causes peripheral bone pain and muscle weakness in adults. In children with atresia of the bile ducts rickets develop. In severe adult cases pseudofractures (Looser's zones) may be seen in the scapula, pelvis, neck of femur and fibula. The condition is best diagnosed, however, from the histological appearances of an iliac crest needle bone biopsy specimen.

Vitamin D 500 000–150 000 units intramuscularly monthly should be given to all patients with prolonged jaundice. Frank osteomalacia is treated initially with weekly injections. Alternatively, the synthetic compounds alfacalcidol (1 $\alpha$ (OH) $D_3$) and calcitriol (1,25 (OH$_2$)$D_3$) are now available, and,

*Pathophysiology and Treatment of Complications* 47

having a shorter half-life in the body, there is less risk of causing hypercalcaemia and renal damage, which can be a serious complication of over treatment with natural vitamin D preparations.

Prophylaxis is with calcium with vitamin D (500 units) capsules daily.

## VITAMIN K

The role of vitamin K is discussed under coagulation disorders (*see* p. 25). It becomes depleted more quickly than vitamin A or D in cholestasis, and then causes prolongation of the prothrombin time (*see* chapter 3).

Deficiency is treated with intramuscular or intravenous vitamin K (phytomenodione) 10 mg daily for 2 days. This should be given routinely to all patients with conjugated hyperbilirubinaemia.

## INFECTIONS

Patients with advanced acute or chronic liver failure are particularly susceptible to infections, and septicaemia is a common cause of death. In the alcoholic there is also an increased risk of pulmonary tuberculosis, and tuberculous and pneumococcal (*Streptococcus pneumoniae*) infections of ascitic fluid may occur.

It is probable that due to venous shunting the liver no longer filters bacteria and bacterial protein from the blood, that immunological defences are reduced, and that leucopenia from hypersplenism all contribute to this increased susceptibility.

## ITCHING

Itching or *pruritus* is a disabling symptom, and is often worse in bed or in the sun. Its aetiology is unknown, although bile acids accumulating in the skin was once thought to be the culprits. It is particularly severe in prolonged cholestasis, such as primary biliary cirrhosis.

### Treatment

Treatment is by advising the patient to use cotton underwear and light bedclothes. Any dryness of the skin is treated with aqueous cream and soap replaced with an arachis oil (Oilatum). Nocturnal hypnotic drugs improve symptoms that are worse in bed.

Cholestyramine (4 g, 2–4 times daily) or colestipol (5 g, 2–4 times daily) are anion-exchange resins and given orally can alleviate itching if cholestasis is not complete.

48 *Chapter 2*

Anabolic steroids are effective. They increase jaundice at the same time, but this may be a small price to pay. Only oxymetholone is now available.

Oral phenobarbitone 60–180 mg nocte has a useful effect, but makes some patients unacceptably drowsy.

Finally, plasmapheresis at 3–4 week intervals can be helpful if drug therapy is ineffective.

## FURTHER READING

Boyer J.L. (1980) New concepts of mechanisms of hepatocyte bile formation. *Physiological Reviews* **60**, 303–26.

Boyer T.D. & Warnock D.G. (1983) Use of diuretics in the treatment of cirrhotic ascites. *Gastroenterology* **84**, 1051–5.

Crossley I.R. & Williams R. (1984) Progress in the treatment of chronic portasystemic encephalopathy. *Gut* **25**, 85–98.

Epstein M. (ed) (1983) *The Kidney in Liver Disease*. 2nd ed. Elsevier, New York.

Fevery J. & Heirwegh K.P.M. (1980) Bilirubin metabolism. *International Review of Physiology* **21**, 171–220.

Heaton K.W. (1972) *Bile Salts in Health and Disease*. Churchill Livingstone, Edinburgh.

Read A.E. (1979). Medical cholestasis. *British Journal of Hospital Medicine* May, 490–7.

Scharschmidt B.F. & Van Dyke R.W. (1983) Mechanisms of hepatic electrolyte transport. *Gastroenterology* **85**, 1199–214.

Wilkinson S.P. (1982) *Hepato-renal Disorders*. Dekker, New York.

Zieve L. & Nicoloff D.M. (1975) Pathogenesis of hepatic coma. *Annual Review of Medicine* **26**, 143–57.

# Chapter 3
# Investigations

## BLOOD TESTS

Investigations of liver disease may involve a number of blood tests being carried out, namely to assess:

Total/conjugated bilirubin
Total bile acids
Serum enzymes
Plasma proteins and immunoglobulins
Coagulation factors
Lipids
Bromsulphthalein retention test
Virological tests
Autoantibodies

### Total/conjugated bilirubin

### BILIRUBIN IN BLOOD

As bilirubin is normally removed from blood only by the liver, its blood level can be used as a true test of liver function. Bilirubin in blood is normally unconjugated and is firmly bound to serum albumin.

Most biochemical methods of measuring bilirubin depend on the diazo reaction described by Paul Ehrlich in 1883. Diazotised sulphanilic acid reacts with bilirubin to give a red colour (azobilirubin) easily measured with a spectrophotometer. This was first used to measure bilirubin in blood by Van den Bergh and Müller in 1912, but Malloy and Evelyn described a reliable method in 1937 and their method, often modified, is still in use.

Conjugated bilirubin reacts *directly* with the diazo reagent, while the unconjugated pigment only reacts *indirectly*, requiring a substance such as methanol or caffeine to accelerate its reaction. Hence by measuring the diazo colour with (total) and without (conjugated) addition of the accelerator, the direct (conjugated) and indirect (conjugated plus unconjugated = total) bilirubin can be measured.

# Chapter 3

---

*Indirect*

$$\text{Unconjugated or conjugated bilirubin} + \text{diazo reagent} \xrightarrow{\text{accelerator}} \text{azobilirubin}$$

*Direct*

$$\text{Conjugated bilirubin} + \text{diazo reagent} \xrightarrow{\text{no accelerator}} \text{azobilirubin}$$

*Therefore*
Indirect − direct value = unconjugated bilirubin
Indirect value = total bilirubin (unconjugated + conjugated)

---

The normal total bilirubin level in blood is less than 17–20 $\mu$mol/litre (1–1.1 mg/dl).

In health, and in disorders of red cell metabolism causing haemolysis, the bilirubin in blood is indirect-reacting or predominantly unconjugated.

The degree of hyperbilirubinaemia is in general a poor guide to the degree of liver cell dysfunction.

## URINE PIGMENTS

### *Urobilinogen*

Urobilinogen in urine is easily detected by adding to urine an equal volume of another Ehrlich's reagent — the aldehyde reagent. The urine turns a pinkish-red colour if an excess amount of urobilinogen is present. This semi-quantitative method is adequate for clinical purposes, though there are methods for extracting the dye and measuring it more precisely.

Two stick tests are available for the semi-quantitative testing of urobilinogen in urine — 'Urobilistix' and 'BM-stix'. Neither are reliable, but nevertheless are much used.

An excess of urobilinogen in urine suggests either:

**1.** an increased hepatic load of bilirubin, such as from haemolysis; or
**2.** mild liver disease. When the enterohepatic circulation of urobilinogen (*see* chapter 2) is impaired, less is extracted by the liver from portal blood, and therefore more circulates in the blood.

## Investigations

### Porphobilinogen

The porphyrin precursor porphobilinogen is excreted in large amounts in the urine in the rare, but dangerous, disease *acute intermittent porphyria*. Porphobilinogen also gives a red colour with Ehrlich's reagent, but can be distinguished from urobilinogen by its different solubility in chloroform; the porphobilinogen colour is soluble in chloroform, but that of urobilinogen is not.

Hence Ehrlich's reagent is added to urine, then a few millilitres of chloroform (and sodium acetate), and shaken. Urobilinogen remains in the upper aqueous layer, while porphobilinogen enters the lower chloroform layer. If there is any doubt at all, send a urine specimen to the laboratory for confirmation *before* permitting anaesthesia or surgery, which can be dangerous in the case of acute porphyria.

### Urobilin

Urobilin in the urine can be detected by its green luminescence when reacted with zinc salts (Schlesinger's reaction), but this test is now obsolete.

### Conjugated bilirubin

Conjugated bilirubin in urine is best detected with the Ictotest tablet. A test tablet is dissolved with a few drops of water on a small paper pad on to which urine has been dropped. A purple colour develops. Unfortunately this test is not sensitive and obviously blood bilirubin levels are more reliable.

The bright colours on filter paper given by Fouchet's test for urinary bilirubin are attractive but obsolete.

The presence of conjugated bilirubin in urine confirms a conjugated hyperbilirubinaemia; it is absent if the blood bilirubin is unconjugated, when there is *acholuric* jaundice, for unconjugated bilirubin does not pass across the renal glomerulus.

## FAECAL PIGMENTS

There are methods for measuring urobilinogen (stercobilinogen) in stool, but they are tedious to perform and the results do not reliably distinguish between intrahepatic and extrahepatic jaundice, for which they were once used. Radiological methods of investigating jaundice have superseded them.

## Total bile acids

Bile acids, like conjugated bilirubin, accumulate in the blood and are excreted in urine when their hepatic excretion is impaired. Being detergents, they lower the surface tension of urine and this was the basis of Hay's test, in which particles of sulphur when sprinkled on urine, and sank if bile acids were present.

Methods for measuring the total and individual bile acids in blood are difficult, although kit tests and radioimmunoassays are now available.

The levels of total or individual bile acids in serum rise early in liver disease, and so fasting levels are a sensitive liver function test. This is especially so after a meal (postprandial) when the bile acids that are stored between meals in the gallbladder are circulating. The test is sensitive because a slight impairment of the uptake of bile acids from the portal blood, coming from the intestine, leads to a relatively large increase of the amount passing through the liver to the systemic circulation. The normal fasting level of total bile acids is up to about 10 $\mu$mol/litre, but the result depends upon the assay method used.

## Serum enzymes

### TRANSFERASES

During liver disease some of the many enzymes in high concentration within liver cells leak across the damaged cell membranes and can be detected in increased amounts in blood. Strictly, these levels in the blood are not measuring the function of the liver, but only indicating its damage.

Two transaminases, which are now called *aminotransferases*, are still the most measured. These are glutamic oxaloacetic transaminase (GOT), now called *aspartate aminotransferase* (AsT), and glutamic pyruvate transaminase (GPT), now *alanine aminotransferase* (AlT). Both are expressed as international units (iu) per litre. AsT is also present in high concentration in skeletal and cardiac muscle, and so its blood level is less specific for liver disease than AlT, but this is not often important.

Normal levels vary from laboratory to laboratory, but are < 20–50 iu/litre. Very high levels of these enzymes, i.e. > 1000 iu, are characteristic of acute hepatitis, but lower levels occur in all types of liver disease and cannot be used to distinguish between them. So raised levels in general only indicate liver disease of some kind.

## λ-GLUTAMYL TRANSFERASE (λGT)

The blood level of the λGT enzyme, also called transpeptidase, has been introduced more recently as a test of liver disease, and is easy to measure. It is also released from damaged liver cells, and so is elevated in similar conditions to those that affect the levels of transferases. Its levels, however, are particularly sensitive to alcohol intake, and are also elevated when hepatic enzyme inducing drugs are ingested, as well as with extrahepatic cholestasis. These responses seem to be due to induction of the synthesis of the enzyme inside liver cells and then its release into the blood, rather than to liver cell damage. The normal level is less than 28 units/litre for men and 18 units/litre for women.

## ALKALINE PHOSPHATASE

The enzyme alkaline phosphatase is present in the liver chiefly in the membranes of bile canaliculi and in bile. Its activity in blood is often increased in liver disease because any local or general obstruction to the flow of bile (i.e. cholestasis; *see* chapter 2) increases its synthesis in the obstructed canaliculi, and increased amounts of enzyme then reflux into blood. It is *not* due to reduced excretion of the enzyme into bile.

An elevated serum phosphatase level is therefore a fairly sensitive test for intrahepatic masses, such as cysts, tumours or abscesses. It is elevated in these conditions before general liver function is affected because the locally obstructed bile canaliculi make more enzyme. It is also often elevated in cirrhosis, and may reach particularly high levels (2–10 times elevated) with intrahepatic and extrahepatic biliary obstruction (cholestasis). Its level does not, however, differentiate between intrahepatic and extrahepatic biliary disease.

Its interpretation is often complicated in bone diseases of growing children by release of the isoenzyme from bone, and in pregnancy the isoenzyme from the placenta. If there is doubt as to the cause of a raised blood level these isoenzymes can be separated semi-quantitatively by electrophoresis. Normal levels vary enormously from laboratory to laboratory depending upon the analytical method used. Thus < 11–13 King Armstrong (KA) units/dl or 90–120 iu/litre are usually normal.

## 5'-NUCLEOTIDASE

An enzyme similar to alkaline phosphatase is 5'-nucleotidase, but it is confined to the liver. Although it is more difficult to measure, elevation of its blood level more specifically indicates liver disease.

54 *Chapter 3*

## Plasma proteins and immunoglobulins

### ALBUMIN

Albumin is synthesised only by liver cells, and is secreted into blood where its half-life time is about 20 days. Severe prolonged impairment of liver cell function therefore lowers its level in blood, although the mechanism of low levels is frequently complex. The level does not fall if the liver damage is recent, such as during the first days of acute hepatitis. It does fall in any patient who is ill with a systemic disease such as an infection, or if the protein is lost in large amounts in the urine or the faeces. So a fall is not specific for liver diseases.

Normal values are about 40–54 g/litre.

### GLOBULIN

Globulins are synthesised by immunocompetent cells throughout the body. Their levels are not reduced by liver disease, and indeed, often increase. This elevation may be due to the immunological disease that is the cause of chronic hepatitis or cirrhosis. It may be because the sick liver allows bacterial and viral antigens to enter the systemic circulation directly from portal blood, i.e. without being removed by the reticuloendothelial, Kupffer's, cells in the liver. In other words they are shunted through and around the liver (*see* portal hypertension, chapter 2). The immunological cells in the body respond to this challenge by synthesising more immunoglobulins, which make up most of the globulin fraction of plasma proteins.

In general, immunoglobulins A and G (IgA and IgG) are elevated in liver disease, but high levels of IgM are particularly characteristic of primary biliary cirrhosis. Measurement of their levels, however, seldom aids diagnosis of liver disease.

These changes of albumin and globulins are the cause of the changes of turbidity and electrophoretic patterns of plasma proteins that were previously used as liver tests but are now obsolete.

### *Caeruloplasmin*

Caeruloplasmin is a globulin that is also a circulating enzyme containing copper. Its levels is markedly decreased in Wilson's disease (*see* chapter 10) due to failure of its synthesis in liver cells.

Normal levels are > 250 mg/litre.

## $\alpha_1 Antitrypsin$ $(\alpha_1 AT)$

$\alpha_1$ Antitrypsin is an enzyme inhibitor in blood the level of which is reduced in several inherited forms (*see* chapter 10). It is associated with neonatal hepatitis, adult cirrhosis and emphysema. Normal levels are about 200 mg/ml.

## $\alpha$ *Fetoprotein (AFP)*

$\alpha$ Fetoprotein is normally present in blood before and soon after birth, but thereafter its concentration falls to low levels. The cells of some tumours, notably primary hepatomata, often begin to synthesise it and its level in blood then rises again. A raised level of fetoprotein suggests the presence of a hepatoma (or choriocarcinoma or teratoma), but it also rises slightly in acute viral hepatitis and pregnancy. Normal levels are less than 10 $\mu$g/litre or 10 MRC units/ml.

## Coagulation factors

Another true test of liver function is the indirect measurement of the amount of the coagulation prothrombin complex factors (II, V, VII and IX) in the blood, since they are synthesised in the liver and have short half-lives in the blood (*see* chapter 2).

Coagulation is measured as the time blood takes to clot in the laboratory after adding a tissue extract and calcium, it is expressed either as the percentage of the normal level of prothrombin activity, or as a prothrombin time (PT) compared to that of a control plasma sample. Thus it is normal if it takes no more than 3 seconds longer to clot than the control, or if the ratio of the time taken a clot of the tested and control plasmas, that is the prothrombin time ratio (PTR), is 1.3 or less.

The prothrombin time is usually abnormal in liver disease for two reasons: first, because of a deficiency of vitamin K, which is obligatory for synthesising coagulation factors in liver cells; secondly, because severely damaged liver cells cannot synthesise adequate amounts of the factors. The time is also abnormal when blood contains inhibitors of coagulation.

After finding an abnormal prothrombin time an intramuscular injection of 10 mg vitamin K is given on two successive days, after which the prothrombin time is measured. The time will return to normal in 48 hours if there is a simple deficiency of vitamin K, perhaps due to intestinal malabsorption of the vitamin (*see* chapter 2), but will not if liver cell damage is the cause.

Since only severe and generalised liver cell damage will reduce the blood

56 *Chapter 3*

level of coagulation factors, the degree of vitamin K resistant prolongation of the prothrombin time is a measure of the severity of advanced liver damage. As it is normal in mild cases, it cannot be used to detect liver disease.

Another coagulation test that can be abnormal in liver disease is the partial thromboplastin time.

## Lipids

The levels of cholesterol and lipoproteins in blood are elevated to prolonged cholestasis, whether intrahepatic or extrahepatic, presumably due to impaired excretion in bile and continued absorption of lipids from food in the intestine. These changes are of no diagnostic value.

Very high levels of cholesterol eventually cause the deposition of cholesterol on skin as raised lumps or xanthomata, and these are particularly characteristic of longstanding primary biliary cirrhosis.

High levels of triglycerides with turbidity of the serum chylomicrons sometimes develop in severe acute alcoholic hepatitis (*see* chapter 9).

### Bromsulphthalein test

A sensitive test of liver function is measurement of the rate of removal from blood of an intravenously administered substance that is chiefly removed from plasma by the liver. Various substances have been tried, such as galactose, but in this country the dye bromsulpthalein has proved convenient and safe. It is easily measured, and the result of the test can be simply expressed as the percentage of the value calculated to be present in the blood at time zero, and that remaining at 45 seconds. So a standard dose of 10 mg/kg body weight is given, and one blood sample taken 45 minutes later. The value at this time is called the percentage retention (normal < 5%). (Figure 3.1)

As an accurate test of liver function, it is abnormal in most cases of cirrhosis. There are many simpler tests and with the increased employment of liver biopsy to diagnose cirrhosis the use of this test has greatly diminished. It is of no value in differentiating the causes of conjugated jaundice, because then it is always abnormal.

### Virological tests

Virological tests are described in chapter 5.

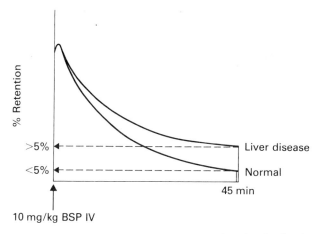

**Fig. 3.1** Bromsulphthalein retention test showing blood levels after intravenous injection of BSP.

## Autoantibodies

A series of so-called tissue antibodies, that is antibodies directed against subcellular fractions of various organs, circulate in some autoimmune chronic liver diseases, and are unusual in the normal population (Table 3.1).

**Table 3.1** Frequency of autoantibodies in autoimmune liver disease.

|  | 'Autoimmune' active chronic hepatitis | Primary biliary cirrhosis |
|---|---|---|
| Antimitochondrial antibody (AMA) | 30% (low titre) | 95% (high titre) |
| Smooth muscle antibody (SMA) | 50% | 50% |
| Antinuclear factor (ANF) | 50% | 20% |

# 58            *Chapter 3*

## ANTIMITOCHONDRIAL ANTIBODY (AMA)

The presence of antimitochondrial antibody diagnostically, is most important. It is almost invariably present in patients with primary biliary cirrhosis (*see* chapter 10). Its absence, therefore, almost excludes this diagnosis. It is, however, also present, but less often and in lower titre, in other types of autoimmune chronic liver disease.

## SMOOTH MUSCLE ANTIBODY (SMA)

Smooth muscle antibody is often present (50%) in the blood of patients with active chronic hepatitis (*see* chapter 8) and, less often, in other autoimmune liver diseases.

## ANTINUCLEAR FACTOR (ANF)

Antinuclear factor may be found in the blood of some patients with severe active chronic hepatitis, as well as in the non-hepatic lupus erythematosis, in which it was first described.

## DIGESTIVE ENDOSCOPY

### Oesophagogastroduodenoscopy

Examination of the upper gastrointestinal tract can be valuable in patients with liver disease. There may be oesophageal and/or gastric submucosal varices, and these are better seen directly with a fibreoptic end-viewing gastroscope than with barium X-rays. At the same time the varices can be injected to sclerose them and prevent bleeding (*see* chapter 2).

Carcinoma of the stomach can be seen and biopsied, while in the duodenum a carcinoma of the ampulla (strictly the papilla) of Vater, or a carcinoma of the head of the pancreas infiltrating the medial wall of the duodenum can be seen and biopsied.

The gastroscopist can detect upper gastrointestinal causes of the bleeding, such as varices, chronic gastric and duodenal ulcers, and acute gastric erosions, which are more common in patients with liver disease.

## ENDOSCOPIC RETROGRADE CHOLANGIOPANCREATOGRAPHY (ERCP)

The extrahepatic and intrahepatic biliary tract can be directly shown in 80–90% of patients by retrogradely injecting radio-opaque contrast material

# Investigations

up through the ampulla of Vater. A long side-viewing fibreoptic duodenoscope is passed into the duodenum, a fine plastic cannula threaded into the papilla and contrast medium injected. Often both the main pancreatic duct system (duct of Santorini) and the biliary tract including the gallbladder can then be seen on X-ray screening, and films taken.

This technique is important when an extrahepatic biliary obstruction, such as a gall stone or pancreatic disease is suspected. It has been perfected over the last 10 years, and is now widely employed. Antibiotic cover may be needed.

A more recent advance has been the technique of cutting open the ampulla with a diathermy wire passed through the duodenoscope, namely *endoscopic sphincterotomy*. This can release gall stones blocking the common duct, or allow a fine wire basket to be passed up to snare and pull the stones down (*see* chapter 16). Indwelling stents can also be placed across bile strictures to allow drainage.

## LAPAROSCOPY

A technique widely used by gynaecologists for examining the pelvis, and used less by British gastroenterologists, involves a laparoscope. This rigid fibreoptic instrument is inserted through the anterior abdominal wall into the peritoneal cavity, which has previously been distended with carbon dioxide. The surface of the liver can be seen and biopsies taken under direct vision, either through the instrument or percutaneously (*see* p. 64). Other organs such as the gallbladder and spleen and the peritoneum can also be seen.

## RADIOLOGY

Radiological investigations of the liver may involve:

> Chest/abdominal plain X-rays
> Barium studies
> Oral cholecystography
> Cholangiography: intravenous, percutaneous and retrograde
> Venography: splenic and hepatic
> Hepatic arteriography
> Liver scans: colloidal, biliary and selenomethionine
> Computed tomography.

### Chest and abdominal plain X-rays

Plain chest and abdominal X-rays can be useful in patients with suspected

60 *Chapter 3*

liver disease. Thus the chest X-ray may reveal a primary bronchial carcinoma or metastases in the lung from an abdominal primary tumour, both of which may have metastasised to the liver and cause jaundice. Pulmonary tuberculosis affecting the liver may be detected. The right hemidiaphragm may be raised when there is a subphrenic abscess above the liver, or an abscess within the liver (*see* chapter 6).

The abdominal X-ray will show the size of the liver and spleen, the presence of calcified gall stones, and any calcified lesions, such as a dead hydatid cyst, within the liver.

Air outlining the biliary tract is seen after passage of a gall stone into the intestine, or when the biliary tract has been anastomosed to the intestine (cholecyst- or choledochojejeunostomy).

### Barium swallow and meal

Oesophageal submucosal varices, a gastric carcinoma, distortion of the stomach by a large liver, or a pancreatic carcinoma distorting the second part of duodenum may be revealed by a barium swallow and meal.

### Oral cholecystography

Filling the biliary tract with a radio-opaque contrast material, oral cholecystography, is only effective if the patient is not jaundiced, for if there is cholestasis the material is not excreted by the liver.

A control plain film is first taken to show any calcified gall stones. Tablets containing a lipid soluble, radio-opaque iodinated material are then taken the night before the main X-rays. The contrast material is absorbed from the small intestine, extracted from the blood by the liver, conjugated in liver cells, and excreted during the night into bile, which collects in the gallbladder. Here it is concentrated by absorption of water across the gallbladder mucosa. The next morning the patient fasts, and plain X-rays and tomograms of the gallbladder are taken with the patient erect and supine. Gall stones show up as filling defects in the dye-filled gallbladder and, depending upon their density, may float or sink as the patient's position is changed.

The patient is then given a small liquid fatty meal to drink. This releases cholecystokinin from the duodenum, and the normal gallbladder contracts, expelling the concentrated material into the common bile duct, which may be opacified. In addition stones may be seen more clearly in the gallbladder when it is contracted and with less contrast material surrounding them.

A second, double dose of contrast material may succeed in opacifying a poorly opacified gallbladder.

# Investigations 61

If no opacification is seen the gallbladder is said to be non-opacified. It is often said to be 'non-functioning', but this is inaccurate as failure to opacify can be due to the patient not taking or vomiting the tablets, or to poor intestinal absorption of the material due to diarrhoea. If these can be excluded, then either the liver cannot excrete the material as in a jaundiced patient, or the gallbladder contains stones that are preventing the material entering the gallbladder through the cystic duct during the night of the test.

This test is, therefore, useless in the jaundiced patient or after cholecystectomy, but it is almost within side effects.

## Cholangiography

### INTRAVENOUS

If the gallbladder has been removed, a similar iodine containing material can be injected or infused intravenously and this is rapidly excreted by the liver into the bile and opacifies the biliary tract, particularly the bile ducts. The opacification, however, is poor, particularly if the patient is jaundiced, and severe anaphylactic reactions to the dye occasionally occur.

This test is therefore much less used now that more direct methods of showing the biliary tract have been developed, namely percutaneous and retrograde cholangiography.

### PERCUTANEOUS

A fine needle with an outer flexible cannula over it is inserted percutaneously into the liver and radio-opaque contrast material directly injected into a small intrahepatic bile duct. In this way it opacifies the biliary tract down to the duodenum. The needle is usually inserted laterally between the ribs. This technique can show the bile ducts even in the deeply jaundiced patient, and is particularly useful in showing the upper margin of a tight bile duct structure.

With a fine Chiba or Okuda needle developed in Japan there is only a small risk of bile leaking along the needle track and causing biliary peritonitis. Bleeding from the liver is another small risk and, as for a needle liver biopsy, the procedure should not be carried out in a patient with abnormal blood clotting or thrombocytopenia without correcting these beforehand. Antibiotic cover is needed.

Percutaneous cholangiography is also performed before the percutaneous insertion of a biliary stent or catheter (*see* chapter 17).

62                                    *Chapter 3*

## RETROGRADE

For endoscopic retrograde cholangiopancreatography (ERCP) *see* p. 58.

### Venography

## SPLENIC

It is sometimes important to opacify the splenic and portal veins, as before performing shunt surgery (*see* chapter 2).

A fine needle is passed percutaneously into the spleen, radio-opaque material injected, and multiple X-rays rapidly taken as the dye passes from left to right across the abdomen in the portal venous system into the liver. The pressure in the splenic pulp can be measured to demonstrate whether portal hypertension is present, and the passage of the dye into the portal veins of the liver, or along abnormal venous collateral vessels, can be documented.

Blood clotting and platelet levels need to be normal for this procedure.

## HEPATIC

A catheter is inserted percutaneously into a brachial or jugular vein and passed through the right atrium into an hepatic vein.

Dye can be injected to demonstrate whether the hepatic veins are patent, and the pressure in the hepatic sinusoids can be measured by 'wedging' the catheter in a small vein. There is then a fixed column of blood from the sinusoids up to the catheter tip and the pressure in the catheter is equal to that in the sinusoids. This is a useful technique in investigating the cause and site of portal hypertension (*see* chapter 2).

A similar technique is used to perform a transjugular liver biopsy (*see* later).

### Hepatic arteriography

A catheter is passed from the femoral artery into the hepatic artery via the coeliac axis and the hepatic arterial vessels opacified with radio-opaque contrast material. This can sometimes be useful in showing the extent of a primary or secondary carcinoma in the liver, or the source of bleeding from the liver. Embolisation of the hepatic arterial blood supply can also be carried out (*see* chapter 11).

The portal vein can be indirectly opacified by injecting dye quickly into the splenic artery and taking X-ray pictures as the dye returns from the spleen and then portal veins.

## Liver scan

There are three methods of showing up the liver by radioisotope scanning (scintiscanning): colloidal, biliary and selenomethionine scans.

### COLLOIDAL SCAN

The most usual liver scan is to inject intravenously a gamma-emitting radionuclide in a colloidal, particulate form. The particles are rapidly removed from blood chiefly by the phagocytic Kupffer's cells in the hepatic sinusoids and by the splenic cells. A technetium colloid is mostly used. The activity in the liver and spleen are then recorded with a gamma counter that scans across the abdomen building up a picture of dots that indicate the local concentration of the particles. Alternatively a rapid picture of the gamma emission from the upper abdomen is taken with a gamma camera — the so-called liver snap.

The scan or snap will show the size of the liver and spleen, and the presence of cold spots, or holes, in the liver from metatases or abscesses more than 2 cm in diameter. A typical patchy appearance of the uptake in the liver is also seen in cirrhosis (*see* chapter 10).

### BILIARY SCAN

A radioactive compound is injected intravenously to obtain a biliary scan and this is taken up and excreted by the parenchymal cells of the liver. The $I^{125}$ labelled dye rose bengal has been used, especially in children with liver disease, and more recently technetium labelled iminodiacetic acid (HIDA) to show the biliary tract has been introduced. The activity of the compounds is seen first in the liver and biliary tract and later in the intestine, and so can be used to demonstrate patency of the biliary tract. The cause of a block, however, is not shown, and the test is not fully reliable.

### SELENOMETHIONINE SCAN

The radioactive amino acid selenomethionine can be used to obtain a scan. This is taken up and incorporated into protein in the liver and the pancreatic cells. Its particular use is to show a primary hepatoma, since the cells of this tumour are able to concentrate the amino acid and thus a 'hole' on a previous technetium scan is filled in. Metatases do not take up selenomethionine and the 'hole' remains.

64 *Chapter 3*

### Computed tomography (CT)

The technique of computing thousands of X-ray tomograms to build up composite transverse pictures through the body has proved useful in the abdomen. The size of the liver and spleen, lesions within the liver, the density of liver tissue, the biliary tract and the pancreas can be shown. Excess iron in the liver in haemochromatosis gives a particularly dense image of the liver.

The technique is safe and not 'invasive' to the patient, but the equipment is expensive and in the UK is available only in a few centres.

## ULTRASONOGRAPHY

B-mode ultrasonography has been greatly developed recently to give good pictures of the liver and biliary tract. The technique is not invasive and is therefore without risk. It will show up intrahepatic lesions, the abnormal structure of the liver parenchyma in cirrhosis, the size of the biliary tract, gall stones, the size and structure of the pancreas, and the size of the spleen. It is particularly good at detecting stonès in the gallbladder, and intrahepatic cysts and abscesses.

## LIVER BIOPSY

Microscopic examination of a small cylinder of liver tissue (*ca.* 2 x 0.3 cm in size or 10–20 mg by weight) is now an important method for diagnosing and planning treatment of diseases of the liver.

### Technique

After local anaesthesia of the skin and subcutaneous tissues in the right mid-axillary line at the upper level of the liver, established by percussion, the biopsy needle is inserted into the liver while the patient holds his or her breath in expiration, and the core of tissue quickly removed. One puncture and specimen are generally sufficient. The patient rests for several hours, initially lying on his or her right side to reduce bleeding from the puncture of the liver capsule. This may involve a stay in hospital overnight, but in some centres it is performed as an outpatient procedure in selected cases.

There is a small risk of bleeding and also, if the biliary tract is obstructed and dilated, of leakage of bile along the needle track into the peritoneum. The prothrombin time and platelet count must be normal, and if not, must be corrected with intravenous clotting factors or platelets. It should not be performed if there is a likelihood of an hydatid cyst or angioma being punctured. The former causes anaphylaxis due to release of the fluid in the cyst,

*Investigations* 65

and the latter bleeding.

It is preferable, if possible, to perform ultrasonography before biopsy to reduce the chances of puncturing a dilated biliary tract that is obstructed or a cyst.

A similar specimen can also be obtained with a special long needle inserted transvenously through a catheter from the jugular vein in the neck via the right atrium and an hepatic vein (transjugular liver biopsy). This can be performed when clotting is abnormal and does not require control of breathing. Also multiple specimens can be obtained.

Percutaneous needle biopsy can be performed under direct vision during laparoscopy (*see* p. 59), when the needle can be directed to a site likely to be positive. Needle and wedge shaped specimens of the liver can also be obtained at laparotomy.

### Histology

The specimen is useful for diagnosing cirrhosis and its causes, e.g. acute and chronic hepatitis, extrahepatic biliary obstruction and tumours of the liver, but isolated local lesions in the liver are easily missed with such a small sample of the organ. Light microscopy, often with special stains, is carried out. Electron microscopy is not useful for clinical work. Wilson's disease (*see* chapter 10) is best diagnosed by measuring the concentration of copper in a specimen of liver tissues.

The rectangular section of the core of liver tissue should include several *lobules*. A lobule (Figure 3.2) is the circular section across a cylinder of tissue around a central vein, that is, the tiniest hepatic vein that joins others eventually to form the hepatic veins. Situated around the edge of this lobule are portal tracts which are small, triangular condensations of reticulin fibres that support a bundle of the smallest tributaries of the hepatic artery, portal vein, bile ducts and lymphatics. Between the portal tracts and central veins are the cords of liver cells, which are arranged in walls one cell thick, rather like canals. Between these walls the blood runs from portal tracts to central veins in the sinusoids, which are lined by fenestrated endothelial cells and flattened reticuloendothelial cells (Kupffer's cells). Outside these lining cells, between them and the liver cells is a space, the space of Disse, into which the cell-free plasma circulates in direct contact with liver cells (Figure 2.3).

Bile canaliculi start as complex invaginations of the cell membranes of two adjacent liver cells, with microvilli projecting into their lumens. These canaliculi combine with others to form bile ductules that pass to the portal tracts. So bile flows towards the portal tracts but blood flows in the opposite direction towards the central veins in the centre of the lobule.

The cords of cells are supported by a network of fine reticulin fibres

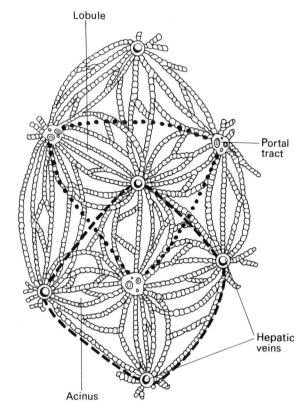

**Fig. 3.2** Microanatomy of the liver. The *lobule* is centred on the central hepatic vein and the *acinus* is centred on the portal tract.

that can be stained with a silver stain (reticulin stain). Any loss of cells causes these fibres to collapse together, *reticulin condensation*.

The portal tracts normally contain only a few leucocytes, and if their number is increased there is said to be inflammation of the tracts. This inflammation can spread out into the lobule areas, the limiting plate of the liver cells surrounding the tract. This is called *aggression*.

An alternative way of considering the microscopic structure of the liver is based on the acinus. This is centred on the portal tract, and round its perimeter are the central veins (*see* Figure 3.2). Functionally it is more logical than the lobule since the blood spreads out from a portal tract towards several central veins, but the concept of the lobule has become more established.

## FURTHER READING

Wright D.G.G. (1983) Liver biopsy. *Hospital Update* **9**, 673–51, 813–26.

# Chapter 4
# Hyperbilirubinaemia and Jaundice

*Hyperbilirubinaemia* is present when the level of bilirubin in the blood is above the normal range. This may be unconjugated and/or conjugated bilirubin. The upper limit of normal values varies between laboratories, but is about 17–20 μmol/litre, or 1.0 mg/100 ml plasma or serum. The level is maximal in the morning.

*Jaundice* occurs with hyperbilirubinaemia when sufficient unconjugated or conjugated bilirubin has diffused into tissues to become clinically obvious first in the sclera and skin. The blood level at which this occurs is about 40–60 μmol/litre plasma or serum.

Jaundice is best classified into three types, namely prehepatic, hepatic and post-hepatic; these are analogous to the three types of uraemia, namely prerenal, renal and post-renal. Older terms such as regurgitant and retention jaundice are confusing and should not be used any longer.

However, it is helpful to divide jaundice (or hyperbilirubinaemia) into two types, depending upon whether the bilirubin in blood is predominantly unconjugated or conjugated, that is > 60% (*see* Tables 4.1 and 4.2).

## UNCONJUGATED HYPERBILIRUBINAEMIA

### Prehepatic

With a greater production of bilirubin due to an increased breakdown of haem, prehepatic unconjugated hyperbilirubinaemia is caused. The liver is able to excrete this bilirubin load, but only when the level in the blood is allowed to rise. This then means that an increased amount of bilirubin is removed per minute from the blood. The plasma hepatic *clearance*, i.e. the volume of blood theoretically cleared of bilirubin, or would have contained the bilirubin, that is removed per minute, remains constant. Compare renal plasma clearance.

There are two main causes (Table 4.1):

**1.** *Ineffective erythropoiesis* — increased ineffective turnover of red cell precursors in the marrow with excess breakdown of haem there.

**2.** *Haemolysis* — increase rate of breakdown of mature red cells and

# Hyperbilirubinaemia and Jaundice

their haem in the circulation by reticuloendothelial cells, chiefly in the spleen and liver.

## CLINICAL FEATURES

Prehepatic hyperbilirubinaemia is characterised by excess unconjugated bilirubin in blood, no bilirubin in the urine (acholuria), an excess of urobilinogen in urine (and faeces), otherwise normal liver blood tests, and often abnormal haematological tests for haemolysis or haemoglobinopathies.

### Liver blood tests

The results of liver blood tests will indicate:

>    Raised serum unconjugated bilirubin
>    Normal enzymes

### Urine tests

In the urine there will be:

>    No bilirubin (acholuria)
>    Excess urobilinogen

### Haemolysis

If there is haemolysis, there will be:

>    Increased reticulocyte count
>    Abnormal haemoglobin electrophoresis
>    Abnormal red cell shapes
>    Increased serum haptoglobin
>    Red cell antibodies
>    Increased red cell osmotic fragility

Jaundice is uncommon in adults with haemolysis since the red cell half-life time in blood has to be very short to increase the bilirubin load enough to elevate the plasma bilirubin level to $> 40$ $\mu$mol/litre (2 mg%), so that jaundice becomes visible.

*Kernicterus*, or brain damage due to raised bilirubin levels, is confined to neonatal jaundice (*see* p. 73). A combination of rapid and abnormal haemolysis before and after birth gives a large bilirubin load, immature conjugating enzymes in the liver, and alteration of the binding of bilirubin to

# 70                                   Chapter 4

albumin. This causes unconjugated bilirubin to diffuse into the brain, particularly the basal ganglia, which *post mortem* may be stained green. Hence kernicterus, or jaundice of the cerebral nuclei, is caused. Hypoxia, acidosis, high levels of free fatty acids (non-esterified fatty acids), and some drugs all contribute to this displacement of bilirubin from its binding to albumin into the brain.

Being lipid soluble, unconjugated bilirubin diffuses across the bowel wall into the lumen, but this is of importance only in the Crigler-Najjar syndrome (*see* p. 72).

Homozygous sickle cell disease (in patients of African origin) and thalassaemia major (in those of Mediterranean origin) are now the commonest causes of severe haemolysis in adults in many UK cities.

Transient unconjugated physiological hyperbilirubinaemia is common in the first 5 days of life (*see* p. 73).

## TREATMENT

Unconjugated hyperbilirubinaemia in the adult is mostly harmless and of cosmetic effect only. Mildly raised levels can be reduced by administering drugs such as phenobarbitone (*see* p. 72), which induce the hepatic bilirubin conjugating enzyme.

### Hepatic unconjugated hyperbilirubinaemia (Table 4.1)

With hepatic unconjugated hyperbilirubinaemia there may be a defect in the uptake of bilirubin by the liver from the blood, or a defect in the storage and conjugation in the liver cells. The rate of excretion of conjugated bilirubin is normal. To overcome this block the level of bilirubin in blood rises, so increasing the gradient from the bilirubin concentration in the blood to that in the liver cells until the steady-state rate of uptake, and then excretion, of bilirubin returns to normal.

Other liver blood tests are normal and there is no excess of urinary urobilinogen, except when the liver defect is combined with haemolysis.

### *Aetiology*

The causes of hepatic unconjugated hyperbilirubinaemia are listed in Table 4.1. A few drugs cause mild hepatic unconjugated hyperbilirubinaemia, notably the antibiotic rifampicin, although the mechanism of its actions on the liver is not clear.

Conjugation of bilirubin in the neonatal liver is immature for some days, and this contributes, together with the excess haemolysis, to neonatal jaundice (*see* p. 73).

# Hyperbilirubinaemia and Jaundice

**Table 4.1** Causes of unconjugated hyperbilirubinaemia

| Prehepatic | Hepatic |
|---|---|
| Haemolysis | Gilbert's syndrome |
| sphcrocytosis | Crigler-Najjer syndromes |
| sickle cell disease | Neonates |
| thalassaemia major | Drugs |
| neonates | rifampicin |
| | |
| Ineffective erythropoiesis | |
| pernicious anaemia | |
| thalassaemia minor | |

The study of congenital defects of conjugation, uptake and reflux of bilirubin by the liver have contributed greatly to our understanding of bilirubin physiology.

## GILBERT'S SYNDROME

Possibly up to 3% of the adult population in the UK normally have levels of unconjugated bilirubin in the blood above 17–20 $\mu$mol/litre (1 mg%), and a few may have up to 100 $\mu$mol/litre. Other liver blood tests are normal, as is the histological appearance of liver biopsy specimens. The bilirubin levels of these patients rise more than is normal during a fast of more than 24 hours, or when they are ill with, for instance, influenza. Such patients are said to have either Gilbert's syndrome, named after a Parisian professor, or benign, constitutional, unconjugated hyperbilirubinaemia.

Many members of their families also have raised bilirubin levels, often not noticed until they are tested. The condition is probably due to several abnormal phenotypes of different genotypes, and is not a simple recessive or dominant characteristic. Hence the results of family studies are confusing.

### Pathophysiology

The mechanism is complex, but includes impaired conjugation and uptake of bilirubin and an increased rate of reflux of bilirubin back into the blood, because its retention inside the liver cell is reduced. In bile there is a greater proportion of bilirubin that has been conjugated with one glucuronic acid

72                                    *Chapter 4*

molecule (i.e. monoglucuronide), rather than the normally predominant diglucuronide.

In addition, in about half these patients the red cell half-life is mildly shortened, and this haemolysis increases the load of bilirubin for the liver and so exacerbates the elevation of bilirubin levels.

## *Diagnosis*

Diagnosis is made by demonstrating raised levels of unconjugated bilirubin in blood without an increased number of reticulocytes, thus excluding severe haemolysis as a cause of the raised bilirubin levels. The liver blood tests other than bilirubin are normal. Haemoglobin electrophoresis may be indicated to exclude an heterozygous haemoglobinopathy, such as thalassaemia minor, which otherwise is easily missed.

Only occasionally is a liver biopsy needed to exclude chronic liver disease. The measurement of the rate of conjugation by a liver biopsy specimen *in vitro* is definitive, but is only a research procedure.

Provocation tests to exacerbate the bilirubin levels more than in normals have been used, such as fasting patients for 48 hours or the intravenous administration of nicotinic acid, but these are seldom needed.

## *Management*

Clinically what must be realised about this harmless condition is that the patients do not have liver *disease*, particularly an extrahepatic obstruction requiring surgery. Abdominal pain from another cause and these raised bilirubin levels can easily suggest gall stones.

Some of these patients may also have difficult obtaining life assurance, since the raised bilirubin levels wrongly suggest chronic liver disease.

No treatment is indicated. Interestingly, the administration of hepatic enzyme-inducing agents such as phenobarbitone and antipyrine lower bilirubin levels. It is not justified, however, to treat a condition that at most gives an abnormal cosmetic effect. The mechanism of this response to drugs may be an increase of the rate of bilirubin conjugation in the liver.

## CRIGLER-NAJJAR SYNDROMES

There are two rare types of Crigler-Najjar syndrome, which are severe, congenital, unconjugated hyperbilirubinaemia caused by defects of bilirubin conjugation in the liver.

*Type I.* There are no conjugates of bilirubin in the bile at all. Some bilirubin diffuses across the bowel into the faeces. The condition is recessively inherited.

*Type II.* Less rare are patients who are less severely affected, and some conjugated bilirubin, chiefly monoglucuronide, is found in bile. This condition may be just a severe form of Gilbert's syndrome. Its inheritance is complex.

In type I, unconjugated bilirubin levels are so high (more than 350 $\mu$mol/litre; 20 mg%) that brain damage, that is kernicterus, invariably occurs. Tragically no treatment is effective, and the bilirubin levels of these patients do not respond to phenobarbitone (*see* Gilbert's syndrome, p. 72).

The bilirubin levels of type II patients do respond to phenobarbitone, but, like patients with Gilbert's syndrome, treatment is seldom justified.

Diagnosis is by demonstrating greatly raised levels of unconjugated bilirubin in blood in neonates (type I) or childhood (type II), and no haemolysis.

## NEONATAL JAUNDICE

Mild transient jaundice in the first 5 days of life is normal or *physiological*, especially in small, premature babies. This is because there is haemolysis soon after birth as the high haemoglobin levels in the fetus falls, adding an extra load to the liver, the conjugating capacity of which is immature for several days.

More extreme jaundice occurs when there is incompatibility of blood groups with a rhesus negative mother and rhesus positive fetus. This is the case particularly if the mother has been sensitised by a previous pregnancy which was similar. Maternal antibodies to the rhesus antigen of fetal red blood cells cross the placenta and attack the cells *in utero* and after birth causing severe haemolysis, anaemia and jaundice (icterus neonatorum).

Neonatal myxodema also causes mild jaundice.

### Treatment

Dangerous levels ($> 350$ $\mu$mol/litre; 20 mg%) in neonates require repeated exchange transfusion of blood via the umbilical vessels to remove the transiently increased pool of bilirubin.

Alternatively phototherapy, in which naked babies are exposed to blue light in an incubator, is often sufficient to prevent the need for exchange transfusion. The bilirubin in the skin capillaries is oxidised and broken down in light to less dangerous and more water soluble products that are quickly excreted into bile.

Finally, phenobarbitone given to mothers (60–120 mg/day) before birth or to the babies themselves also reduces bilirubin levels and can be tried.

74 *Chapter 4*

## CONJUGATED HYPERBILIRUBINAEMIA

The condition of conjugated hyperbilirubinaemia includes all patients with general medical and surgical disorders of the liver. Bilirubin conjugates predominate in blood and are excreted in urine. The urinary excretion prevents enormous levels of bilirubin occurring in blood, except when there is concomitant renal failure. Thus plasma levels above 500 μmol/litre (30 mg%) are unusual.

The patient may notice dark urine (from excreted conjugates) and pale stools (no degraded pigments excreted in faeces) (*see* chapter 2), and itching may occur. There are *hepatic* and *posthepatic* causes (Table 4.2).

**Table 4.2**   Causes of conjugated hyperbilirubinaemia

| Hepatic | Posthepatic or extrahepatic |
|---|---|
| Without cholestasis<br>    Dubin-Johnson syndrome<br>    Rotor syndrome<br><br>Cholestasis<br>    acute or chronic hepatitis (*chap.* 5–8)<br>    cirrhosis (*chap.* 10)<br>    intrahepatic tumours (*chap.* 11)<br>    lymphomata (*chap.* 13)<br>    jaundice of pregnancy (*chap.* 14)<br>    sclerosing cholangitis (*chap.* 18)<br>    intrahepatic biliary atresia (*chap.* 18) | Gall stones (*chap.* 16)<br>Carcinoma of pancreas (*chap.* 17)<br>Chronic pancreatitis (*chap.* 17)<br>Carcinoma of bile ducts (*chap.* 17)<br>Extrahepatic biliary atresia (*chap.* 18) |

## Hepatic

### CONGENITAL CAUSES

There are two rare conditions in which conjugated bilirubin is present in the blood, but otherwise patients are well. Jaundice presents in young adults.

## Hyperbilirubinaemia and Jaundice

### *Dubin-Johnson syndrome*

In cases of the Dubin-Johnson syndrome, the liver is black when looked at by laparotomy or laparoscopy, as is a needle liver biopsy specimen. This strange appearance is due to an accumulation of black pigments in the liver, presumably from a defect in the excretion into bile of precursors of the pigment.

Bilirubin levels in blood are usually less than 90 $\mu$mol/litre (5 mg%). There is a defect in the excretion of bilirubin conjugates into bile, and of iodine containing radio-opaque compounds, so a cholecystogram usually fails, hence these patients often undergo unnecessary cholecystectomy. Other biliary constituents are not retained, and so there is no cholestasis.

### Rotor syndrome

A rare group of similar patients have nearly the same syndrome, but the liver is not black and this is known as the Rotor syndrome.

### ACQUIRED CAUSES

Acquired causes of hepatic conjugatged hyperbilirubinaemia include medical diseases of the liver (*see* Table 4.2). A better term is *intrahepatic cholestasis*, since this emphasises blockage of the flow of bile (*see* chapter 2).

### Posthepatic

Posthepatic conjugated hyperbilirubinaemia is often termed *obstructive* jaundice, but the word obstructive is confusing and best not used. Extrahepatic cholestasis is a better term. Other terms are extrahepatic or surgical jaundice, since all lesions involving the extrahepatic biliary tract are included in this group, and most are amenable to surgical treatment.

### Neonatal

Jaundice continuing after the first few days of life is uncommon. It may be due to atresia of the intrahepatic or extrahepatic ducts (*see* chapter 18) or to neonatal hepatitis.

### NEONATAL HEPATITIS

Hepatitis may be due to infections, such as congenital rubella, toxoplasmosis or bacterial sepsis. The cause of some cases of neonatal hepatitis is obscure,

76  Chapter 4

and the liver then may contain giant multinucleated cells (giant-cell hepatitis). One-third of these children die.

There are also rare familial syndromes of neonatal intrahepatic cholestasis.

## INVESTIGATION OF THE JAUNDICED PATIENT

Few patients should now have to undergo diagnostic laparotomy without the surgeon knowing at least that the jaundice is definitely due to extrahepatic cholestasis, and preferably knowing the exact site of the obstruction of the biliary tract.

The central decision to reach is the differentiation between intrahepatic (medical) and extrahepatic (surgical) causes of cholestasis. There is, however, seldom urgency in coming to a decision in the diagnosis of jaundice, and it is usually better to wait and perform or repeat investigations rather than gamble with the patient's condition. This is unlike the management of renal disease, when relief of postrenal obstruction is urgent. One exception is bacterial cholangitis, which may require urgent surgical drainage to control septicaemia, but even here modern antibiotics are temporarily effective.

### Unconjugated hyperbilirubinaemia

First exclude unconjugated hyperbilirubinaemia in every jaundiced patient. Although an uncommon cause of frank jaundice (*see* p. 68), it must not be mistaken for cholestasis from disease of the liver or biliary tract.

There is no dark urine (i.e. acholuric jaundice), pale stools nor itching. The bilirubin in blood is predominantly unconjugated, and if there is haemolysis there is an excess of urobilinogen in the urine (Ehrlich's test or stix tests). Other liver blood tests are normal. There may be other haematological abnormalities, such as a raised reticulocyte count and abnormal haemoglobin electrophoresis.

### Conjugated hyperbilirubinaemia

Provided that cholestasis has been established (dark urine, pale stools, itching) only one disease, namely acute viral hepatitis, can sometimes be managed without investigation, but only if the history, physical signs and routine blood tests *strongly* indicate this. Then all that needs to be done is to watch the patient's recovery carefully.

In all patients, or if recovery from the presumed hepatitis is not rapid, the following investigations are mandatory:

# Hyperbilirubinaemia and Jaundice

1. Routine haematology, for haemoglobin level, red cell size and white cell and platelet counts.
   Routine liver blood (function) tests: bilirubin, alkaline phosphatase, one aminotransferase (aspartate or alanine), and albumin levels.
   Prothrombin time (or ratio).
   Hepatitis B surface antigen and hepatitis A IgM antibody.
   Chest X-ray and plain abdominal X-ray.
   These tests will only diagnose with certainty some cases of acute viral hepatitis, i.e. if they have very high transferase levels > 500 iu/l. Some other tests (*see* below) are therefore added, where appropriate.
2. Conjugated/unconjugated bilirubin fractions.
   Gamma glutamyl transferase level.
   Paul-Bunnell test.
   $\alpha$ Fetoprotein level.
   Ultrasonography.
   If this indicates that the biliary tract is not dilated, i.e. intrahepatic jaundice is likely, then further tests are carried out.
3. A scintiscan of the liver and/or a liver biopsy is performed. If ultrasonography suggests dilated ducts, gallstones, or a pancreatic lesion, then either percutaneous or retrograde cholangiography is carried out. The expertise of the local hospital staff may dictate which of these two is first carried out, but, for instance, a suspected lesion of the pancreas favours retrograde cholangiography.
4. If these tests show that the dilatation or obstruction of the biliary tract suggested on ultrasonography is *not* present, then a liver scintiscan and/or biopsy is carried out.
   In this way an appropriate cause of almost all cases of jaundice of patients should be diagnosed within 2 weeks of admission to hospital.

## FURTHER READING

Axon A.T.R. (1979) Approach to the jaundiced patient. *British Journal of Hospital Medicine* May, 464–77.
Bouchier I.A.D. (1981) Diagnosis of jaundice. *British Medical Journal* **283**, 1282–4.
Brodersen R. (1980) Bilirubin transport in the newborn infant, reviewed with relation to kernicterus. *Journal of Pediatrics* **96**, 349–56.
Editorial (1978) Hereditary jaundice. *Lancet* **2**, 926–7.
Editorial (1979) Diagnosis of cholestasis. *British Medical Journal* **1**, 1232.
Johnson J.D. (1975) Neonatal nonhemolytic jaundice. *New England Journal of Medicine* **292**, 194–7
Popper H. Cholestasis. *Hepatology* **1**, 187–91.

78 *Chapter 4*

Read A.E. (1979) Medical cholestasis. *British Journal of Hospital Medicine* May, 490–7.

Valman H.B. (1980) Jaundice in the newborn. *British Medical Journal* **280**, 543–5.

Vennes J.A. & Bond J.H. (1983) Approach to the jaundiced patient. *Gastroenterology* **84**, 1616–18.

# Chapter 5
# Acute Viral Hepatitis

Acute hepatitis is inflammation and destruction of the parenchymal cells of the liver that lasts no more than 6 months. If the hepatitis lasts longer than this, then it is by convention termed *chronic* hepatitis.

The commonest cause of acute hepatitis is a viral infection, but other causes are bacterial infections (*see* chapter 6), reactions to drugs (*see* chapter 7), and alcohol excess (*see* chapter 9). The time course of symptoms and liver blood tests for viral hepatitis are given in Figure 5.1.

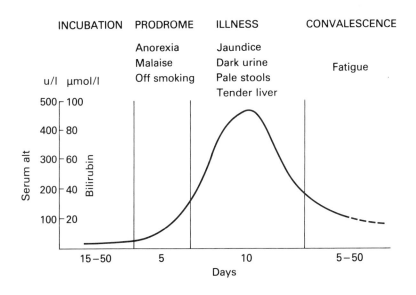

**Fig. 5.1** Time course of symptoms and liver blood tests in viral hepatitis.

Many viruses invade and damage the liver; some are listed in Table 5.1. At least three viruses, A, B and non-A, non-B, are liver specific or *hepatotropic* (*see* p. 84) having a special affinity for liver cells.

80 *Chapter 5*

**Table 5.1** Viruses that invade and damage the liver

| | |
|---|---|
| Hepatotropic viruses | Hepatitis A (HAV)<br>Hepatitis B (HBV)<br>Non-A, non-B viruses |
| Other viruses | Epstein-Barr (glandular fever)<br>Ricksettsia burnetti (Q fever)<br>Cytomegalovirus<br>Herpes simplex<br>Rubella virus<br>Yellow fever<br>African viruses<br>    Lassa fever<br>    Rift Valley fever<br>    Marburg virus |

## SYMPTOMS

All hepatitis viruses may produce similar prodromal symptoms, that is symptoms before jaundice appears, these include:

> lethargy
> anorexia and nausea
> distaste for smoking or alcohol
> arthralgia
> rashes

Malaise, anorexia and nausea are frequent. Many patients lose even previously strong addictions to smoke and to drink alchol.

With hepatitis B infection, arthralgia (pains in the joints), less commonly arthritis (pains plus swelling and tenderness of joints), and skin rashes can occur before the jaundice.

Right-sided upper abdominal and lower thoracic discomfort is frequent. Frank pain may be severe and mimic pain from the biliary tract, presumably due to stretching of the capsule of the liver. Mild diarrhoea may be noticed, and fever, sweats and even occasionally rigors.

Many patients remain anicteric (without jaundice) and may never be diagnosed, the infection remaining subclinical.

After a few days, however, most patients become jaundiced. This is usually mild and lasts no more than 1–2 weeks, but occasionally is severe and prolonged. The urine becomes dark and the stools pale, i.e. there is cholestasis.

## Recovery

Recovery is usually rapid. The patient starts to feel better, appetite returns, the urine becomes less dark and finally clinical jaundice fades.

Quite a few patients feel lethargic and depressed for weeks or even months after viral hepatitis (*posthepatitis syndrome*), just as they may after any virus infection such as influenza. These patients need to be strongly reassured that they will eventually completely recover.

After recovery the patient is immune to that particular type of hepatitis, but not to other viruses.

The overall mortality of viral hepatitis is less than 1%. Fulminant liver failure (*see* chapter 2) is rare but develops when damage to the liver is rapid and severe (Figure 5.2). Death follows in a third of these. Bruising, hepatic encephalopathy and ascites are ominous signs. Recovery can occur even from coma, and then is usually complete.

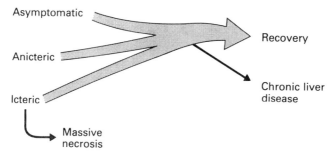

**Fig. 5.2** Clinical types of hepatitis and possible outcomes.

In a few patients with hepatitis B or non-A, non-B, low grade liver damage continues for months or years after the initial illness. After about 6 months the hepatitis is termed chronic, and it may progress to cirrhosis (*see* chapter 8).

Hepatitis B can also cause an autoimmune syndrome of polyarteritis, with widespread vasculitic damage to the skin, joints, kidney and nerves.

## EXAMINATION

Examination may reveal jaundice, scratch marks, and in fulminant cases, bruising. The liver is usually enlarged, smooth and tender on palpation and percussion. The spleen becomes palpable in a few. Ascites is unusual.

Asterixis (flap) and hepatic fetor develop in the few with fulminant liver failure.

82                          *Chapter 5*

## INVESTIGATIONS

A typical case does not always require biochemical investigation, but if there is any doubt about the diagnosis, and there usually is, and also to reassure the patient, a few simple tests are indicated.

### Urine

Conjugated bilirubin is present in the urine before jaundice appears and persists until the jaundice has almost disappeared. Urobilinogen may also be present in excess at the beginning of the illness, but testing for this is unreliable.

### Blood count

The level of haemoglobin should be unaffected. The white cell count is often reduced, and atypical mononuclear cells may appear. Occasionally haemolytic or aplastic anaemia occur. The sedimentation rate is often normal (sic).

### Liver blood tests

The bilirubin in blood is conjugated. Levels above 100 $\mu$mol/litre (5 mg%) are unusual.

The serum alkaline phosphatase level is usually only slightly elevated, to about twice normal. If cholestasis is prolonged the level may become much more elevated and then falsely suggest extrahepatic cholestasis.

Typically, aminotransferases (transaminases) at first are greatly elevated to ten times normal, or even to 1–5000 units/litre. But levels rapidly fall and may be much lower or even normal by the time the patient presents to the doctor. The level is a poor guide to the severity of the disease. Slightly abnormal levels may persist for months (transaminitis) as part of the posthepatitis syndrome (*see* p. 81).

Gamma-glutamyl transferase levels will also be elevated.

The prothrombin time becomes prolonged in severe (fulminant) hepatitis, due to liver cell failure, and suggests a poor prognosis. In prolonged cholestasis, however, lengthening of the prothrombin time can be due to malabsorption of vitamin K, the fat-soluble vitamin that is required for the hepatic synthesis of some clotting factors (*see* chapter 2).

Albumin levels only fall if the disease is prolonged and severe, but are often non-specifically depressed in the elderly.

Immunoglobulin levels increase, but this is of no value in diagnosis.

### Virological tests

For a discussion *see* p. 85.

### Liver biopsy

It is sometimes, but not usually, necessary to perform a percutaneous needle biopsy of the liver if the diagnosis is in doubt, such as when cholestasis is prolonged. The prothrombin time and platelet count need to be normal to minimise the risk of bleeding.

During the early phase of acute viral hepatitis parenchymal cells throughout the hepatic lobules die, especially those around the central veins, and there is infiltration of the liver with inflammatory cells. Afterwards regeneration is usually complete. If the necrosis is severe and the reticulin framework collapses, damage may extend across from one central vein to a portal tract, called *bridging necrosis*. This is associated with a poorer prognosis. During the cholestatic phase bile plugs, that is tiny yellow-brown plugs of debris in the biliary canaliculi, are seen and are presumed to be inspissated bile.

Hepatitis B virus can be detected in sections of liver by staining with orcein, or by immunofluorescence with sera containing antibodies to the surface or core antigens (*see* p. 87). Some infected cells also have opaque cytoplasm (ground-glass cells).

## MANAGEMENT OF VIRAL HEPATITIS

### Diagnosis

Liver blood tests should be performed in any patient suspected of having developed hepatitis, and serum hepatitis B surface antigen and hepatitis A antibodies looked for (*see* pp. 85 and 87).

In a young adult who gives a clear history of contact with another patient with hepatitis, and has prodromal symptoms and greatly elevated serum transferase levels, the diagnosis is simple. But such cases are now unusual. So if there is any doubt, and the patient does not rapidly improve, further tests such as ultrasound, liver biopsy or direct cholangiography (percutaneous or retrograde) should be performed (*see* p. 58). The less usual causes of viral hepatitis (Table 5.1) should be considered.

84                                    *Chapter 5*

## Treatment

There is still no specific treatment for viral hepatitis. Most patients can be managed at home, particularly if there is a spouse or relatives to care for them.

Bedrest is advised while the patient is jaundiced and feels wretched, but not essential. Physical activity should be moderate. A low fat diet is often recommended, and although it is not necessary, some patients do feel nauseated eating fatty foods. Otherwise a normal diet is recommended.

Corticosteroids cause the jaundice to disappear more quickly, but are not advised since they do not really help and they may increase the chances of the virus persisting in the liver and thus causing chronic hepatitis and cirrhosis.

Alcohol should be forbidden for a few weeks only, although there is no evidence that in moderation it is toxic.

Patients are often worried that they may infect their family, but, by the time they present to the doctor, usually they are becoming less infectious, particularly with hepatitis A. At home the patient should be careful with toilet hygiene to reduce faecal-oral transmission, and should carefully remove any blood if he or she cuts the skin. There should be no sharing of toothbrushes. Hepatitis B can be spread sexually but the risk of infection is low unless the patient's blood remains positive for hepatitis B and the 'e' antigen (*see* p. 88). A sheath is best worn during sexual intercourse.

Any person who has had hepatitis is never allowed to donate blood.

In hospital, care should be taken with faeces and blood specimens, but rigorous barrier nursing is not indicated. Contact with infected blood should be minimised by the wearing of gloves by nurses, doctors etc. if their skin is broken by cuts or eczema. Gloves, however, make venepuncture more difficult and do not protect against the possible puncture of the skin by a needle contaminated with blood.

There is no treatment for posthepatitis lethargy except firm reassurance; but antidepressant drugs and nocturnal hypnotics can be useful. Corticosteroids are not recommended.

## HEPATOTROPIC VIRUSES

There are at least three, and probably more, viruses that primarily attack the liver, as opposed to those viruses that produce disease of other organs while also affecting the liver. These are hepatitis A, B and non-A, non-B viruses.

## Hepatitis A

### EPIDEMIOLOGY

The incidence of hepatitis A has been falling in the UK from 23 500 in 1970 to 3200 in 1979 (England and Wales). Although it is now rising, only a minority of the population are immune. It is maximal in the winter. Hepatitis A virus causes what was once called infectious hepatitis, since it is highly infectious and spreads easily in epidemics by the faecal-oral route, especially when personal hygiene is poor. It is more frequent in non-immune visitors to tropical countries, while in the past there have been large epidemics in the armed forces.

The incubation period is 3–4 weeks. The disease usually occurs in children and young adults, and in homosexuals. It is a mild illness, and death is rare. It is not followed by chronic hepatitis, but prolonged lethargy can occur after recovery. It is not transmitted parenterally, that is by transfusion of infected blood or blood products, but occasionally sexually.

### VIROLOGY

The cause of hepatitis A is a small (27 nm diameter), ribonucleic acid enterovirus. It has recently been identified in faecal specimens by electron microscopy and has been grown in the laboratory.

The virus is excreted in the faeces especially during the prodromal period. Excretion is less once jaundice appears, and infectivity then becomes low.

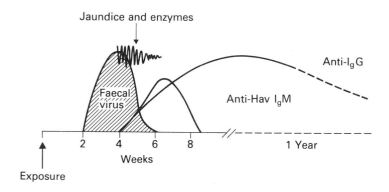

**Fig. 5.3** Virological and serological results during the course of hepatitis A.

86 *Chapter 5*

The presence in the blood of rising titres of antibodies to the virus can now be used to make a firm diagnosis of hepatitis A. Immunoglobulin M (IgM) antibodies last only 2–3 months and their presence therefore indicates recent infection, while IgG antibodies persist for years (Figure 5.3), and may only indicate infection long past and immunity to re-infection.

The virus and its antigen and antibody are now abbreviated to HAV, HAAg and anti-HA, respectively.

## PROPHYLAXIS

An intramuscular injection of gamma globulin (immune serum globulin, ISG) 0.02–0.12 ml/kg gives good passive protection against hepatitis A and is advised for those travelling to tropical countries, or for close contacts of patients. It is effective up to 14 days after exposure, but protection only lasts 6 months. It is best to check before administration, that the patient is not already immune, i.e. already has serum anti-HA antibodies present.

## Hepatitis B

Previously called serum hepatitis (or homologous serum hepatitis), hepatitis B (HB) often followed injections of pooled serum obtained from several donors, one of whom was carrying the hepatitis B virus.

## EPIDEMIOLOGY

Hepatitis B is increasing in the UK, and now constitutes about half of all reported cases of acute hepatitis. It can be transmitted by blood, or products obtained from blood, such as plasma, factor VIII concentrate etc, both from infusions and through contaminated needles ('needle-stick'). It can probably be transmitted sexually, also possible by biting insects, and certainly from a mother to her baby during delivery (misnamed 'vertical' transmission, but not strictly *in utero*).

It is more frequent in males than females and in homosexuals, drug addicts, multiply transfused patients such as haemophiliacs, renal dialysis patients, patients in long-term institutions, and in residents of tropical countries and Greenland. Medical personnel and dentists have a slightly increased risk.

It is not as easily transmitted as hepatitis A, requiring to be directly inoculated through skin or mucous membrane.

## CLINICAL

The disease is in general less mild than hepatitis A and carries a higher mortality, but this is still less than 0.5%. Prodromal features such as arthralgia and skin rashes can be a feature.

The virus may persist in the liver for years after an attack (the *carrier state*) and probably therefore for life, presumably because the immune system is unable to react fully against it. It may then cause varying degrees of chronic hepatitis, cirrhosis (*see* chapter 8), and hepatoma (*see* chapter 11).

All these patients are at risk of transmitting the disease by donating blood. Medical attendants can contract it from accidental needle puncture of their skin by a contaminated needle ('needle-stick'), such as during surgery or dentistry.

Hepatitis B virus is occasionally found in the blood of patients with polyarteritis, which is thought to be caused by antigen-antibody complexes.

## SERUM MARKERS

The hepatitis B virus was first detected in 1965 as an antigen in the blood of an Australian aboriginee, when sera from multiply transfused American patients reacted *in vitro* against his blood. It was therefore called Australian antigen, later hepatitis associated antigen (HAA), and now hepatitis B surface antigen (HBsAg), with several other antigens and antibodies (*see* p. 88).

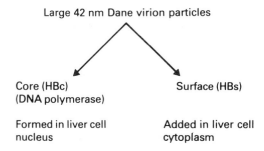

**Fig. 5.4** Main components of hepatitis B virus.

### *Virus particle*

With the electron microscope three types of particle can be seen in the serum of patients with hepatitis B (Figure 5.4). These are the large *Dane particle* (42 nm diameter) which is the complete virus made up of a 27 nm core of deoxyribonucleic acid, an *inner coat* containing the core antigen (HbcAg) and 'e' antigen (HbeAg), and a *surface coat* containing protein and the surface antigen (HBsAg). There are also in blood much higher numbers (up to $10^{13}$/ml) of spherical and tubular particles that are derived from the protein, lipid and carbohydrate surface. It is thought that the infectious viral core multiplies and causes the liver cells to add the protein coat, perhaps to protect the core against the host's immunological attack.

*Antigens*

Routine testing for hepatitis B detects the antigen derived from the surface of the particle (HBsAg), but antibodies (anti-HBs and anti-HBc) can often also be detected in serum (Figure 5.5). In addition the 'e' antigen (HbeAg) can sometimes be detected, in which case the enzyme DNA polymerase (DNAp) and Dane particles are usually present in blood. When the 'e' antigen, DNAp and whole virus particles are present, the serum of the patient is highly infectious. Later the antibody to 'e', anti-HBe usually appears.

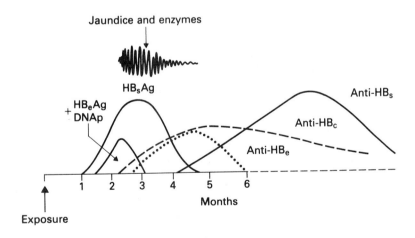

**Fig. 5.5** Virological and serological results during a course of hepatitis B infection.

There are at least ten subtypes of HBsAg that are of epidemiological interest.

A new antigen, delta antigen, has been found in some patients with chronic hepatitis B, and is associated with a superimposed attack of acute hepatitis. It is another tiny opportunistic virus.

## Time course on serum markers

During the prodromal phase of hepatitis B the first serological marker to appear is HBsAg 2–8 weeks before the clinical illness and about 4 weeks after exposure. This is followed by HBeAg and DNA polymerase, their presence indicating whole virus particles in the serum, and hence high infectivity. HBcAg may appear briefly at this time when jaundice is at its peak. The antibodies to HBsAg, HBcAg and HBeAg then appear and infectivity rapidly decreases as the titre of HBsAg falls. Usually the final marker is anti-HBs antibody, which when present alone indicates a previous infection and immunity against further attacks of hepatitis B, but not of other viruses.

In about 10% of patients contracting hepatitis B, the virus persists in the liver for more than 6 months and tests for viral antigens in the serum remain positive — the so-called *carrier* state (Figure 5.6). At first the virus is extrachromosomal in the liver cells where it replicates and causes the cells to synthesise large amounts of HBsAg, which is secreted into the blood. Free virus is present in the blood, HBeAg is detected, and the patients are highly infectious. Prolonged liver damage may occur, namely chronic hepatitis (*see* chapter 8) and cirrhosis, and later hepatoma.

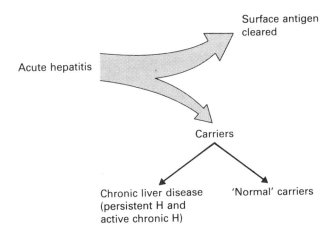

**Fig. 5.6**  Virological outcomes of infection with hepatitis B.

Over the next few years the virus integrates with the liver cell's own DNA, free virus and HBeAg disappear from blood, and infectivity is reduced. The risk of hepatomata developing remains (*see* chapter 11), and HBsAg remains positive. Liver damage is now usually mild or absent unless it has already progressed to cirrhosis, when it is irreversible.

90 *Chapter 5*

## PROPHYLAXIS

Normal immune serum globulin (ISG) does not contain sufficient antibody to hepatitis B virus to offer much protection, but hyperimmune globulin (HIG) collected from donors with a high titre of these antibodies is partially effective.

An injection of 0.5–0.7 ml of ml/kg is therefore given to hospital personnel as soon as possible after an accidental needle prick, and repeated 1 month later, and to contacts of patients with acute hepatitis. A smaller dose is given to infants within 2 days of being born to mothers carrying the virus, especially if they are HBeAg positive. The number infected by the virus from their mothers can thereby be reduced. Those spouses of patients with acute or chronic hepatitis B who do not have anti-HBs should also be immunised.

Recently a major advance has been the preparation of vaccines from hepatitis B particles isolated from serum. These vaccines have been shown in high risk groups (homosexuals, patients on renal dialysis) to give excellent active protection against acquiring the disease. They are becoming available to hospital personnel and other exposed subjects, such as dialysis patients and spouses of chronic carriers, but at the moment cost precludes their use in developing countries where hepatitis B is such a scourge. They have not been shown to be effective if administered after inoculation of the virus.

## MANAGEMENT OF THE CARRIER

Carriers need reassurance since there is no means of removing their virus. Simple precautions against shared toothbrushes and razors, and with spilt blood are continued. The virus can probably be transmitted sexually. It is difficult to reassure heterosexuals and homosexuals when one partner is not yet infected, although vaccine should be offered. It is possible to advise against promiscuity and to advise mechanical protection. Those with 'e' antigen, sometimes called *supercarriers* are particularly dangerous. Close family members, particularly babies at birth, are also at risk. If liver blood tests are normal or near normal, then they are unlikely to develop serious chronic liver disease.

### Non-A, non-B hepatitis

Features of non-A, non-B hepatitis:

> Caused by unidentified virus(es)
> Chiefly parenteral transmission
> Generally mild acute hepatitis

20% followed by chronic hepatitis and cirrhosis
Autoantibodies negative
No specific treatment

Serological testing has shown that only one-third of post transfusion hepatitis was due to hepatitis B, which is now almost excluded by testing donor blood, and so the remaining two-thirds are termed non-A, non-B hepatitis. It now accounts for more than three-quarters of post transfusion hepatitis in the United States. Many cases, however, are sporadic and not associated with transfusion.

The incubation period is variable, usually 6–10 weeks. The acute hepatitis is usually mild, but is followed by mild to severe chronic liver disease in about 20% of patients. Probably several viruses will eventually be shown to be involved, but none has yet been properly characterised.

## NON-HEPATOTROPIC VIRUSES

### Epstein-Barr virus

The Epstein-Barr virus, which causes infectious mononucleosis or glandular fever, can also cause an acute hepatitis. This is usually subclinical, but jaundice can occur. A positive Paul-Bunnell test should give the diagnosis, and there are circulating atypical mononuclear cells.

### Q fever

Q fever is clinically similar to Epstein-Barr virus.

### Cytomegalovirus

Cytomegalovirus is transmitted in blood and can cause hepatitis and jaundice, particularly in immunologically impaired patients such as after renal transplantation and cardiac surgery. Serum antibody titres rise and the virus may be found in urine.

### Herpes simplex and rubella

Herpes simplex and rubella cause hepatitis in infancy.

92    *Chapter 5*

## Yellow fever

The yellow fever virus still causes severe epidemics in South America and Africa. It is due to an arbor virus transmitted by mosquitos from monkey to man. Severely affected patients die with a bleeding diathesis; jaundice develops only in survivors.

## Other tropical viruses

Lassa fever, Rift Valley fever and Marburg virus diseases cause hepatitis in Africa.

## Hepatitis in pregnancy

*See* chapter 14.

## Postoperative hepatitis

*See* chapter 7.

## FURTHER READING

Bowen E.T.W. & Simpson D.I.H. (1981) Dangerous virus diseases. *Hospital Update* **7**, 175–85.
Dienstag, J.L. (1983) Non-A, non-B hepatitis. *Gastroenterology* **85**, 439–62.
Editorial (1984) Passive and active immunoprophylaxis of hepatitis B. *Gasteroentology* **86**, 958–81.
Sherlock, S. (ed) (1980) Virus hepatitis. *Clinics in Gastroenterology* **9**, No 1.
Zuckerman, A.J. (1981) Acute viral hepatitis. *Journal of the Royal College of Physicians* **15**, 88–94.

# Chapter 6
# Bacterial and Parasitic Infections

### BACTERIAL HEPATITIS

Bacteria, like viruses, can invade liver cells and cause acute hepatitis. But they never cause chronic hepatitis.

### Septicaemia

Septicaemia is frequently accompanied by abnormal liver blood tests, and liver biopsy reveal infiltration of the lobules and portal tracts by polymorphonuclear white cells. Jaundice is unusual.

### Leptospirosis

A sometimes serious infection, leptospirosis is now uncommon in the UK with 61 confirmed cases in 1982, but it still causes a few deaths (4 in 1982). It is contracted from rats, chiefly by agricultural and sewerage workers, coal miners etc. There are several spirochaetes that cause different forms of the disease. The *Leptospira icterohaemorrhagiae* subgroup causes the severest form, called Weil's disease, with jaundice and bleeding due to the hepatitis, and also renal failure.

After incubation for 1–2 weeks there is a high fever and prostration with a peripheral polymorphonuclear leucocytosis, and at this time the spirochaetes can be detected in the blood by microscopy. The course of the infection is shown in Table 6.1.

Jaundice, proteinuria, meningitis and skin bruising develop, and the bacteria appear in urine. Finally, improvement may occur as the serum antibody titre rises.

There is no specific treatment, although penicillin is recommended.

### Syphilis of the liver

*Congenital* fibrosis of the liver and cirrhosis are now rare. They followed invasion of the liver by the spirochaetes *in utero*. *Secondary* syphilis is associated with a mild hepatitis when the spirochaetes damage the liver.

94 *Chapter 6*

**Table 6.1** Course of leptospirosis

| Incubation | First week | Second week | Third week |
| --- | --- | --- | --- |
| 1–2 weeks | Septicaemia<br>    headaches<br>    back pains<br>    fever<br>    spirochaetes<br>      in blood | Hepatitis<br>    jaundice<br>    purpura<br>    bruises<br><br>Nephritis<br>    proteinuria<br>    spirochaetes<br>      in urine<br>    uraemia<br><br>Meningitis<br>    meningism<br><br>Leucocytosis | Recovery<br>    serum antibody<br>    titres rise |

*Gummata*, as part of the chronic, *tertiary* phase of syphilis, are now rare. Treatment is with penicillin.

### Tuberculosis of the liver

Tubercle bacilli frequently invade the liver in systemic tuberculosis. When liver blood tests are abnormal in a patient with suspected pulmonary tuberculosis but sputum is negative, histological and bacteriological examination of a needle liver biopsy specimen is a good means of detecting the bacilli. Granulomata with caseating centres and acid-fast bacilli are found scattered in the hepatic lobules; occasionally jaundice occurs.

Treatment is with rifampicin and isoniazid for up to a year, and ethambutol for 6–8 weeks.

## LIVER ABSCESS

Necrosis of an area of liver cells leads to an abscess, which may coalesce with others to form larger, loculated intrahepatic masses. They are either pyogenic, that is caused by bacteria, or amoebic, caused by *Entamoeba histolytica*.

## Pyogenic

A pyogenic liver abscess may occur up to several years after an abdominal operation, or may be caused by bacterial cholangitis from gall stones (*see* chapter 16), or occur spontaneously without cause. The organisms are usually gram negative, and recently anaerobic and carbon dioxide requiring species such as *Bacteroides* and *Streptococcus milleri*, which are difficult to culture in the laboratory, have predominated.

### CLINCAL FEATURES

The onset may be abrupt with a swinging fever, sweats, rigors, jaundice and right hypochrondial pain, or more gradual. The liver is enlarged and tender to palpation and percussion, and over it there may be a peritoneal rub usually in inspiration (*see* chapter 1), and a right pleural effusion.

A liver abscess is a not-to-be-forgotten cause of a fever (pyrexia) of unknown origin (PUO).

### INVESTIGATIONS

As with all intrahepatic mass lesions, liver function tests show an elevated alkaline phosphatase, mildly raised aminotransferase levels, and later jaundice. There is a peripheral polymorphonuclear leucocytosis.

Percutaneous needle aspiration of the pleural effusion reveals white cells in the fluid or frank pus, and repeated blood cultures are often positive. The diaphragm may be elevated on chest X-ray, and occasionally 'tented' up, as a suprahepatic or subphrenic collection of pus develops under it. An isotopic liver scan will show the filling defect(s), as will ultrasonography, which will also often detect fluid within the abscess or gall stones when they are causing the underlying cholangitis.

### TREATMENT

Treatment always used to be surgical, with the insertion under general anaesthesia of a percutaneous drain, but now percutaneous aspiration and precise antibiotic treatment can often cure. Large abscesses should be aspirated with a long needle, preferably guided by ultrasound, and as much pus as possible aspirated. This is then examined microscopically and cultured.

Antibiotic treatment is tailored to the organism found and should last for at least 4 weeks. The size of the lesions as they shrink can be conveniently and safely followed by repeated ultrasound examinations and

96 *Chapter 6*

aspiration as necessary.

Surgery is indicated if abscesses do not rapidly resolve.

### Amoebic

In tropical countries the protozoon *Entamoeba histolytica* can invade the bowel wall to cause colitis, and then less often spread via the portal blood to the liver. Here they slowly kill groups of liver cells and cause abscesses. The body reacts poorly to the organisms and there is no true pus, that is no collection of polymorphonuclear leucocytes, in the abscess. The liquefied liver cells retain a pink colour and supposedly look like anchovy sauce.

## CLINICAL FEATURES

The patient has usually travelled in an endemic area within the previous few months, and often has been living 'rough', but occasionally the onset is delayed by many years.

Symptoms are more gradual than with a pyogenic abscess, with weight loss, lassitude, right hypochrondrial pain that is worse on inspiration, sweats, and relatively mild fever. There may also be pain felt in the right shoulder tip referred from the diaphragm. The liver is tender on palpation, and sometimes there is right hypochrondrial rub on inspiration.

A right pleural effusion and a raised right diaphragm may be found. Before treatment became effective, it was not rare for the untreated abscess to rupture through the 'tented' diaphragm into the lung so that the 'pus' was dramatically coughed up!

## INVESTIGATION

Jaundice is unusual, but the serum alkaline phosphatase level is elevated and there is anaemia and mild polymorphonuclear leucocytosis. The active, vegetative form of the parasite can often be found in a recently passed stool, in fresh rectal mucus obtained at sigmoidoscopy, and in biopsy specimens of the rectal mucosa. In the rectal mucosa they form deep, flask-shaped ulcers as they dissolve their way into the mucosa.

If the bowel alone is involved, serological tests (e.g. fluorescent antibody test) are often negative, but they always become positive when the liver is invaded. So a negative test excludes hepatic amoebiasis, but a positive test only makes it possible.

A chest X-ray may reveal the raised, sometimes 'tented', diaphragm, and a pleural effusion. An isotope liver scan or ultrasonography will show the abscess.

## TREATMENT

Treatment used to be with emetine, which was effective but toxic to the heart, or chloroquine. However, now metronidazole 800 mg tds for 5–10 days is used. It is safe and effective, and also treats the bowel infestation, although it does sometimes cause nausea, particularly if alcohol is ingested concomitantly.

At the same time, larger abscesses should be aspirated percutaneously with a needle, preferably with ultrasound guidance. Large quantities of 'pus' can be removed, and the patient rapidly improves.

Surgery is now rarely indicated.

## PARASITE INFESTIONS

### Malaria

Except when patients are extremely ill with malignant (*Plasmodium falciparum*) malaria, liver damage by these protozoa does not occur. Jaundice and centrilobular necrosis of liver cells is then probably due to shock and poor perfusion of the liver.

In malarious areas liver biopsy specimens frequently reveal excess iron in the reticuloendothelial Kupffer's cells, and this is due to chronic haemolysis

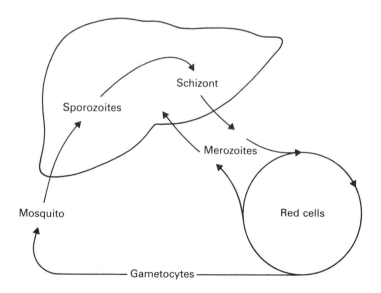

**Fig. 6.1** Life cycle of a malarial infection.

98 *Chapter 6*

releasing iron from damaged red cells ingested by the Kupffer's cells. Although malarial sporozoites invade liver cells and later release merozoites into the blood (Figure 6.1), this does not cause much liver damage. The liver maintains the relapsing cycles of tertian (*P. vivax*) and quartan (*P. malariae*) malaria by harbouring the intermediate merozoite forms.

Immunological reactions to chronic infection with malaria may be the cause of the obscure *tropical splenomegaly syndrome* in Africa. Marked splenomegaly develops with portal hypertension and oesophageal varices but liver function and histology are preserved.

## TREATMENT

Treatment is with chloroquine or quinine, plus primaquine to clear the liver of *P. vivax*.

### Leishmaniasis

In tropical countries invasion of the liver and spleen by the protozoan *Leishmania donovani* causes visceral, as opposed to cutaneous, leishmaniasis. There is chronic fever, and the spleen is greatly enlarged, the liver less so. The organism is seen within macrophages in these organs and sometimes in the bone marrow.

## TREATMENT

Treatment is with pentavalent antimony (stiboglu conate 600 mg daily by injection for 4 weeks).

### Hydatid disease

The tapeworm *Echinococcus granulosus* lives in the intestine of the dog, and man becomes a futile intermediate host by ingesting the cysts in canine excreta contaminating salads etc. (Figure 6.2). Sheep do likewise, and in them the cycle can then be maintained when the dogs eat the viscera of the dead infected sheep. Hence hydatid disease is rare in towns, but more common in rural, sheep-farming areas, such as Wales, the Eastern Mediterranean and Australasia.

In man, the outer layer of the ovum is digested by the stomach. The liberated ovum burrows through the intestinal wall and reaching the liver in portal blood, slowly grows there over years into an adult cyst that eventually may contain thousands of young scolices. Less often ova reach the lungs or brain and produce a cyst there. The growing cyst excites little

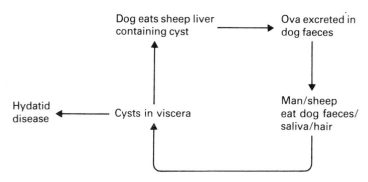

**Fig. 6.2**   Life cycle of a hydatid infection.

inflammatory or immunological response and is surrounded only by compressed liver cells. Many cysts die and calcify.

## CLINICAL FEATURES

Calcified dead cysts are detected as a round, radio-opaque ring or as amorphous streaks on plain abdominal X-ray. Many cysts are silent and thus detected by chance X-rays, at surgery, or *post mortem.*

Hepatomegaly may be found, and this can cause an hypochondrial aching pain. Cysts can rupture into the biliary tract, and then become infected and cause a pyogenic abscess, or rupture into the peritoneal cavity when multiple new cysts are seeded. Occasionally the cysts grow and spread within the liver and cause jaundice.

## INVESTIGATIONS

Peripheral blood eosinophilia may be present, and the serum alkaline phosphatase level is elevated. Isotope liver scan or ultrasonography delineate the cyst(s).

If the cyst has leaked, immunological hypersensitivity may occur. This may be detected by a wheel and flare after intradermal injection of hydatid fluid (Casoni test), but otherwise there are accurate serological tests.

## TREATMENT

No treatment is needed if there are no complications; otherwise surgery is required. Alcohol is first injected into cysts to sterilise the contents and then they are carefully removed without rupturing and spilling the contents.

100 *Chapter 6*

The drug mebendazole is worth trying. Albendazole has recently been tried with success.

## Schistosomiasis

Infestation by trematodes (flukes) occurs in tropical countries, and hepatic involvement is chiefly due to *Schistosoma mansoni* and *japonicum*, rather than *haematobium*, which usually affects only the urinary bladder.

In man the eggs are excreted from the intestine in the faeces. They hatch in water and their embryos enter the intermediate host, a water snail, and develop into cercariae. These then penetrate naked human skin exposed to water and travel in the blood stream to the intestine and/or bladder. The adult worms develop in the intrahepatic veins and migrate down into the mesenteric veins where they lay eggs. These are carried back to the liver and lodge in the portal tracts, where they excite a chronic foreign body reaction. The local fibrosis slowly obliterates the portal vein radicles, and the flow of portal blood into the liver is progressively reduced so that a presinusoidal portal hypertension develops (*see* chapter 2). A true cirrhosis, however, does not follow. Some eggs work their way through the intestinal wall and are excreted.

### CLINICAL FEATURES

The liver and spleen initially enlarge, but later the liver may shrink. Gastro-oesphageal varices due to the portal hypertension cause gastrointestinal bleeding, and ascites and oedema develop. As there is no damage to the liver cells and no cirrhosis, liver function is preserved and jaundice does not occur. Hypersplenism may cause a normocytic anaemia, leucopenia and thrombocytopenia.

The stool of rectal biopsy specimen may contain the ova, and a liver biopsy specimen will show ova in portal tracts in the centre of granulomata and local fibrosis.

### TREATMENT

Schistosomiasis is often treated with antimony compounds, but newer drugs are more effective, though more toxic. Niridazole (12.5 mg/kg bd for 5–7 days) is effective but is dangerous in patients with portal hypertension because the drug is then shunted around and through the liver directly to the systemic circulation without being detoxified, causing encephalopathy. The antimony compound, stibocaptate, which is given intramuscularly (8 mg/kg for 5 days) is less toxic.

# Bacterial and Parasitic Infections

Praziquantel, however, is now the best drug (4 mg/kg as a single oral dose).

The usual treatment for bleeding varices is required, although as liver function remains good and there is no cirrhosis, these patients do well after endoscopic sclerosis or shunt surgery (*see* chapter 2).

## Liver flukes

### SHEEP LIVER FLUKES

Invasion of the liver by the sheep fluke *Fasciola hepatica* occurs in rural areas, such as Wales in the UK. Eggs are passed from the bile ducts by sheep into their faeces, and these become mobile and penetrate a mud snail. Cysts formed by the mobile metacercariae are discharged from the intermediate snail host and are then ingested by man on wild watercress or similar leaves. In the intestine the parasite escapes from the digested cyst and penetrates the bowel wall, reaching the liver by crossing the peritoneum, i.e. not in the blood stream. In the liver they pass to the bile ducts.

Some months later fever, rigors, weight loss, cough and pruritis develop. The liver is enlarged and tender. There is eosinophila and raised alkaline phosphatase. This is the picture of cholangitis. Some days later ova can be found in the faeces.

#### Treatment

Treatment is with bithionol, or more recently praziquantil or nicbofan, but is disappointing. Most patients slowly recover.

### CHINESE LIVER FLUKE

In the Far East *Clonorchis sinensis* is ingested in raw fish. It prefers the larger bile ducts in which it causes chronic infection with cholangitis, gall stones, fibrosis and, in a minority, primary carcinoma of the small bile ducts, *cholangiocarcinoma* (*see* chapter 17). There is eosinophilia.

#### Treatment

Treatment of the infection is either with bithionol, but this is unsatisfactory, or is chiefly surgical.

102 *Chapter 6*

## FURTHER READING

Editorial (1980) Pyogenic liver abscess. *British Medical Journal* **280**, 1155–6.

Morris D.L. (1981) Management of hydatid disease. *British Journal of Hospital Medicine*, June, 586–95.

Neoptolemus J.P. & Macpherson D.S. (1981) Pyogenic liver abscess. *British Journal of Hospital Medicine* July, 47–55.

Perera M.R., Kirk A. & Noone P. (1980) Presentation, diagnosis and management of liver abscess. *Lancet* **2**, 629–32.

Peters R.S., Gitlin N. & Libke R.D. (1981) Amebic liver abscess. *Annual Review of Medicine* **32**, 161–74.

# Chapter 7
# Drug and Toxic Hepatitis

Since so many drugs are removed from blood by, and concentrated in liver cells and then metabolised and thereby usually detoxified, is not surprising that they or their metabolites sometimes cause damage to the liver. Drugs metabolised in liver cells are usually oxidised, the so-called *phase I*, and then conjugated, *phase II*, with amino acids or sugars before they are excreted into bile.

Although the distinction is becoming blurred, it is still convenient to consider drugs and chemicals causing hepatitis as either *predictable* or *unpredictable* hepatotoxins.

## PREDICTABLE ACUTE HEPATOTOXINS

Drugs and chemicals that at different doses invariably and predictably cause liver damage in man and animals are known as predictable acute hepatotoxins. The damage may be caused by the primary drug molecule or by its metabolites, and so the rate of metabolism of one to the other is crucial. This explains why the hepatotoxic dose per kg body weight varies widely from species to species, and why the toxicity of a drug may be altered by hypoxia or by pretreatment with drugs that either induce or inhibit microsomal enzymes in the liver.

Histologically, cell damage is variable and may be maximal either in the periportal or centrilobular regions of the liver lobules.

Some drugs that can cause hepatitis include:

paracetamol
tetracycline
carbon tetrachloride
mushrooms
yellow phosphorus
Epping poison
ferrous salts
tannic acid

All are rarer causes of an hepatitis than viruses or alcohol.

104 *Chapter 7*

## CLINICAL FEATURES

The clinical picture is similar for all. After a delay of 1–3 days when the patient feels relatively well, nausea, vomiting, jaundice with greatly raised levels of aminotransferases, and an enlarged tender liver develop and then subside over the next 1–2 weeks with complete recovery.

With larger doses, jaundice is followed by prolongation of the prothrombin time, bruising, encephalopathy, and occasionally death from acute hepatic necrosis.

The clinical picture therefore closely resembles acute viral hepatitis. Histologically, too, the appearances are similar or identical. Cirrhosis does *not* ever follow a single episode.

### Paracetamol

In 1970 there were 29 deaths in England and Wales out of 890 hospital admissions for large overdoses (> 15 g) of paracetamol, chiefly taken with suicidal intent. By 1977 there were 144 deaths. Women aged 20–30 predominate.

After such an overdose, an early stomach washout may remove unabsorbed tablets, and oral administration of charcoal is given to bind unabsorbed toxin and slow its absorption. Blood levels of paracetamol are measured.

Recent work on the mechanism of paracetamol hepatotoxicity has shown that increasing the supply of sulphur-containing amino acids to the liver cells enables more of the drug to be combined with gluthathione and hence inactivated. So, if the blood paracetamol levels are high, oral methionine (2.5–4 g, up to 4 times hourly) and intravenous acetylcysteine (150 mg/kg over 15 minutes) are now given as soon as possible. If given early enough they reduce liver damage and mortality.

If liver damage occurs, treatment is as for viral hepatitis (*see* chapter 5).

### Tetracycline

Liver failure occurred after large intravenous doses of tetracycline especially in pregnancy, but is now rare. The drug is particularly toxic to the kidney and liver in patients with preceding renal and liver failure. Histologically, the liver cells show striking infiltration with tiny vesicles of fat, and is related in some way to inhibition of protein synthesis in liver cells by the drug.

### Carbon tetrachloride

Although used to produce liver damage in laboratory animals, this is rarely ingested by patients.

### Mushroom poisoning

A few *Amanita* species contain hepatotoxins that can cause delayed death from liver and renal failure, but cases in the UK are rare. It is commoner in Continental Europe and the United States.

### Yellow phosphorus

Yellow phosphorus is ingested in fireworks by children, chiefly in France and South America.

### Epping jaundice

In 1965 in the Epping area of North London an hepatotoxin was inadvertently incorporated into bread and caused an epidemic of jaundice.

### Ferrous sulphate

Overdoses of iron tablets can cause acute gastritis and liver damage. Their colour attracts children.

### Tannic acid

Tannic acid added in barium enemata to improve the coating of the mucosa of the colon used to cause liver damage, but lower safe concentrations are now used.

## PREDICTABLE CHOLESTASIS

Anabolic steroids (i.e. C17 substituted steroids) and oestrogens always impair to some extent the excretion of substances into bile, and so they cause mild cholestasis. Jaundice, however, is rare except in pregnancy (*see* chapter 14).

106                        *Chapter 7*

## UNPREDICTABLE ACUTE HEPATOTOXINS

Eight per cent of adverse drug reactions reported to the Committee on Safety of Medicines involved liver damage, and the number of drugs reported to do this, and the number of cases, are increasing. Every drug should be therefore assumed occasionally to cause liver damage. Some drugs which have been known to cause liver damage include:

> monoamine oxidase inhibitors
> antituberculous drugs
> methyldopa
> oral hypoglycaemic drugs
> antithyroid drugs
> some antibiotics
> sulphonamides
> phenylbutazone
> phenytoin

Sometimes only one or two doses of drug seems to be sufficient, and so a careful drug history is mandatory in any jaundiced patient. It may be necessary to check the drug history with the patient's doctor. However, more usually the drug has been taken for several days or more.

### Unpredictable acute hepatitis

### CLINICAL FEATURES

Usually unpredictable acute hepatitis is mild, and may only be noticed from abnormal liver function tests, particularly raised levels of aminotransferases. It usually rapidly remits on withdrawal of the drug, but occasionally fulminant liver failure and death occur. Less often the picture of cholestasis develops with jaundice, itching and raised alkaline phosphatase levels, but normal or near-normal aminotransferase levels. This may persist for months.

Histologically the liver shows varying degrees of inflammation, sometimes eosinophils being prominent, with necrosis of liver cells, or cholestasis with little inflammation but bile plugs in biliary canaliculi. Granulomata can be a feature.

The mechanism of these reactions is unknown, since only a few can be reproduced in animals. There is increasing evidence that individuals are susceptible because of genetic differences in rate or type of metabolism of the particular drug in their liver cells.

## REPORTING

Every suspected case of drug-induced liver damage in the UK should be reported to the Committee on Safety of Medicines, 1 Nine Elms Lane, London SW8, on special yellow postcards. Only in this way can an unusual sporadic adverse effect of a drug be established.

### Monoamine oxidase inhibitors

Monoamine oxidase inhibitors are the most likely to cause severe liver damage relative to the frequency of their administration.

### Antituberculous drugs

Mainly rifampicin and isoniazid, antituberculous drugs frequently cause transient mild elevation of aminotransferases that decline with continued treatment. Higher levels (> 300 iu/litre, or elevated up to ten times), however, indicate that the drugs must be withdrawn, because progressive liver failure can occur.

Rifampicin also causes a benign, mild unconjugated hyperbilirubinaemia. The patient should be asked quickly to reattend if nausea, vomiting, dark urine or jaundice are noticed.

### Phenothiazine

Phenothiazines, especially chlorpromazine, are the commonest cause of cholestasis due to drugs. Occasionally this can be prolonged for months, but more usually rapidly recovers.

### Management

Since most patients rapidly improve when the drug is withdrawn, they are best managed conservatively without invasive investigations, as for viral hepatitis. But when the cause of the jaundice is unclear the usual management of the jaundiced patient is needed, with direct cholangiography and/or liver biopsy (*see* chapter 3).

The trial re-administration of a suspected hepatotoxin is too dangerous to be recommended.

108           *Chapter 7*

## POSTOPERATIVE JAUNDICE

### Halothane

Mildly abnormal liver function tests are frequent following anaesthesia and surgery, but jaundice is uncommon, and liver failure and death rare. This reaction is more common when halothane is administered within 1 month after a preceding exposure, and in obese patients.

Halothane probably more frequently causes liver damage than other anaesthetic agents, but the statistics are debated. It is a safe agent and therefore is more widely used than others. The mechanism of the toxic reaction is uncertain, but probably involves the metabolism of halothane in liver cells, perhaps precipitated by hypoxia of the liver cells due to the hypotension and reduced liver blood flow induced by anaesthesia. There is evidence also of a transient immunological hypersensitivity to liver cells components in patients after an episode of postanaesthesia liver damage.

Clinically, a transient fever follows the operation and precedes the jaundice, but this can, of course, be due to other postoperative causes. Liver dysfunction is not noticed until jaundice appears between the third and seventh day. Recovery is usually rapid, but occasional patients deteriorate and die with liver cell failure.

The choice of anaesthetic agent after previous recent anaesthesia, or after previous postoperative jaundice depends on judging between the anaesthetic advantages of halothane and the risks (medical and legal) of liver damage. Each case must be individually assessed by the anaesthetist.

### Postoperative cholestasis

Postoperative cholestasis can follow cardiac operations (post-pump jaundice) and may be related in some way to poor hepatic perfusion during prolonged bypass surgery. It can improve spontaneously, but is generally associated with a poor outcome.

## POST-TRANSFUSION JAUNDICE

Viral hepatitis due to B or non-A, non-B hepatitis viruses follows 2–3 months, and sometimes much more, after transfusion of infected blood.

Haemolysis of transfused blood and of blood in tissues after surgery causes increased bilirubin production and contributes to an unconjugated jaundice in the first days after surgery, and also exacerbates jaundice due to liver damage.

## Drug and Toxic Hepatitis

## UNPREDICTABLE CHRONIC HEPATITIS

Drugs are an occasional cause of an unpredictable chronic hepatitis (*see* chapter 8) and cirrhosis. If it is suspected, they should be withdrawn. Conversely, a careful drug history is mandatory in patients with chronic liver disease.

### Oxyphenisation

Oxyphenisation is a laxative drug that can cause chronic hepatitis when taken for long periods. It has now been withdrawn from the market.

### Methyldopa

Methyldopa uncommonly causes liver damage, but often haemolysis.

### Aspirin

Aspirin has recently been noted frequently to cause abnormal liver blood tests and a mild chronic hepatitis in patients with rheumatoid arthritis taking large doses for a prolonged period. It is reversible.

## UNCONJUGATED HYPERBILIRUBINAEMIA

Unconjugated hyperbilirubinaemia may be predictable or unpredictable. Sulphonamides compete with bilirubin for its binding to albumin, and thereby increase tissue bilirubin levels and jaundice. This is of importance only in the neonate (*see* kernicterus, chapter 4).

Many drugs occasionally cause haemolysis and mild unconjugated hyperbilirubinaemia (e.g. methyldopa, sulphonamides). Some antibiotics, notably rifampicin, fucidin and novobiocin, can cause a harmless hepatic unconjugated jaundice.

Drugs can also predispose to hepatomata (*see* chapter 11), to vascular abnormalities of the liver (*see* chapter 12) and to gall stones (*see* chapter 16).

## FURTHER READING

Collins J.D., Bassendine M.F., Ferner F., Blesovsky A., Murray A., Pearson D.T. & James O.F.W. (1983) Incidence and prognostic importance of jaundice after cardiopulmonary bypass surgery. *Lancet* **1**, 1119–23.

Davis M. (1980) Drug-induced disorders of the liver. *British Journal of Hospital Medicine* July, 17–23.

110 *Chapter 7*

Editorial (1980) The Liver and halothane. *British Medical Journal* **280**, 1197–8.

Keeling P.W.N. & Thompson R.P.H. (1979) Drug-induced liver disease. *British Medical Journal* **1**, 990–3.

Prescott L.P. (1983) Paracetamol overdosage. *Drugs* **25**, 290–314.

Timbrell J.A. (1983) Drug hepatotoxicity. *British Journal of Clinical Pharmacology* **15**, 3–14.

# Chapter 8
# Chronic Hepatitis

Inflammation of the parenchymal liver cells, namely hepatitis, lasting more than 6 months is termed *chronic hepatitis*. So jaundice or abnormal liver function tests for more than 6 months plus the histological appearances of a liver biopsy specimen establishes the diagnosis. If less than 6 months, it is still an acute hepatitis (*see* chapter 5).

There are two types: *persistent (chronic) hepatitis* (PCH) also called chronic persistent hepatitis (CPH), and *active chronic hepatitis* (ACH) also called chronic active hepatitis (CAH) or chronic active liver disease (CALD). They are differentiated by the histological appearances of the liver biopsy specimens (Table 8.1), and the progression of ACH to cirrhosis.

### AETIOLOGY

Strictly, histological chronic hepatitis can be caused by the following diseases:

> Autoimmune disease
> Hepatitis B
> Hepatitis non-A, non-B
> Inflammatory bowel disease
> Unpredictable hepatotoxic drugs
> Chronic, destructive, non-suppurative cholangitis (primary biliary cirrhosis)
> $\alpha_1$-antitrypsin deficiency
> Wilson's disease
> (Alcoholism)

Alcohol is usually thought of as causing acute hepatitis and subsequently cirrhosis (*see* chapter 9), even though a chronic hepatitis must always precede cirrhosis.

# Chapter 8

## PERSISTENT CHRONIC HEPATITIS

### CHRONIC HISTOLOGY

In the portal tracts there is a mild degree of inflammation, that is, infiltration with chronic inflammatory mononuclear cells, chiefly lymphocytes. These cells do not spread across the limiting plate of cells into the lobules, which remain normal (Figure 8.1). There is no fibrosis nor cirrhosis.

### AETIOLOGY

Persistent hepatitis is found in about a third of chronic carriers of hepatitis B virus, and about 40% of patients after suffering from non-A, non-B hepatitis progress to chronic persistent hepatitis. A transient, self-limiting persistent hepatitis may also follow hepatitis A.

Alcohol (*see* chapter 9) and a few drugs (*see* chapter 7) can cause the histological features of persistent hepatitis, which also occur in patients with severe inflammatory bowel disease (ulcerative proctocolitis and Crohn's disease).

### CLINICAL FEATURES

After an attack of viral hepatitis some patients remain mildly ill, with lassitude, anorexia, depression and a right hypochondrial ache. Liver blood tests are mildly abnormal, with slightly raised blood levels of bilirubin, which may be unconjugated, of aminotransferases and of gamma glutamyl transferase. Serum albumin, alkaline phosphatase and prothrombin time are normal.

Other patients present to the doctor with abnormal liver blood tests, but without a preceding history.

Histological examination of a needle liver biopsy specimen reveals the diagnosis.

### TREATMENT

As described in chapter 5, provided hepatitis B virus is not present the only treatment needed is reassurance of the patient that the condition will spontaneously improve. Corticosteroids are not advised. Sometimes antidepressant drugs are needed for a period.

In a few of these patients this lesion will progress to cirrhosis, and so in general it is benign. Even those with persistent hepatitis due to chronic carriage of the hepatitis B virus only infrequently progress to acute chronic hepatitis.

# Chronic Hepatitis

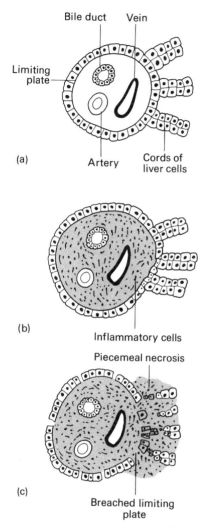

**Fig. 8.1** Normal portal tract (a); persistent hepatitis with increased inflammatory cells within the portal tract (b); and aggressive hepatitis with cells eating out into the lobule (c).

114 *Chapter 8*

## ACTIVE CHRONIC HEPATITIS

### HEPATIC HISTOLOGY

With active chronic hepatitis, there is an *aggressive* hepatitis, in which the central parts of the lobules are spared, but the periportal areas are infiltrated with chronic inflammatory cells spreading out from portal tracts across the limiting plate. Some of the periportal parenchymal cells are like islands, surrounded by inflammatory cells and later by fibrosis, and eventually they die — so-called piecemeal necrosis (Figure 8.1).

If the condition progresses cirrhosis develops, and so these appearances are not benign. The combination of periportal inflammation and cirrhosis is then termed an *active cirrhosis* or alternatively, active chronic hepatitis with cirrhosis.

### AETIOLOGY

The condition of active chronic hepatitis was first recognised in young women who had circulating lupus erythematosus cells (LE cells), and was therefore called lupoid hepatitis. However, such patients are a minority, and this term should be abandoned to avoid confusion with a quite separate disease, systemic lupus erythematosus, which rarely affects the liver.

Apart from some of the diseases listed in Table 8.1, there are two main groups of patients with active chronic hepatitis: hepatitis B virus (HBV) negative patients and hepatitis B virus positive patients. These patients are without or with the hepatitis B surface antigen (HBsAg) or other HBV markers in blood.

**Table 8.1**  Description of histological appearance of chronic hepatitis

| Persistent chronic hepatitis | Active chronic hepatitis |
| --- | --- |
| Inflammation localised to portal tracts | Aggressive inflammation invading lobules |
| No cirrhosis | Cirrhosis frequent |
| Liver function tests mildly abnormal | Hepatitis B unusual |
| Hepatitis B frequent cause | Corticosteroids beneficial |
| Corticosteroids not indicated | Prognosis variable |
| Good prognosis | |

## Chronic Hepatitis

### Hepatitis B negative ('autoimmune') active chronic hepatitis

Features of autoimmune chronic hepatitis are given in Table 8.2. This disease has a higher incidence in women. There are circulating immunological markers such as lupus erythematosus (LE) cells in 15% of cases, antinuclear factor (ANF) and smooth muscle antibody (SMA) in 50%, antimitochondrial antibody (AMA) in low titre in 30%, and rheumatoid factor (RF) in 20%.

**Table 8.2**    Autoimmune chronic hepatitis

Hepatitis B virus negative
Women > men
Autoantibodies frequent
Other autoimmune diseases often present
Responds to corticosteroids

### AETIOLOGY

The predominance of women, the association with other immunological diseases, the presence of circulating antibodies, the histological appearance of the liver, the response to corticosteroids, and the frequency of HLA antigens (*see below*) all suggest this is an immunological disease. It may be triggered, however, by an initial virus infection, or there may be a continuing infection by some unidentified non-A, non-B virus.

More careful testing for markers of hepatitis B virus other than the surface antigen (HBsAg), such as anti-HBc (core antibody), has revealed that some cases are due to covert chronic infection with this virus (*see* chapter 5).

### CLINICAL FEATURES

The disease may present with jaundice, sometimes after a previous episode of jaundice that initially seemed to resolve completely. In other cases the disease may be less severe particularly in older patients when abnormal liver blood tests lead to a diagnostic liver biopsy being performed.

The signs and symptoms of an established cirrhosis may be present early. Weight loss and malaise are frequent, as is amenorrhoea. Spider naevi, palmar erythema, acne and hirsutes occur in younger women, and gynaecomastia in men. The liver is usually enlarged and may be tender.

116 *Chapter 8*

Splenomegaly, ascites and oedema, and oesophageal varices may develop.

Involvement of other organs by immunologically based diseases is common. Arthralgia and, less commonly, swelling and arthritis of the fingers, wrists and knees may be present. Diabetes, thyrotoxicosis, renal tubular acidosis, glomerulonephritis, the sicca syndrome (dry eyes), and pulmonary fibrosing alveolitis all occur more frequently than expected.

Liver blood tests confirm conjugated hyperbilirubinaemia, raised levels of aminotransferase enzymes, sometimes as high as in acute hepatitis (viz > 1000 iu/litre), only slightly raised alkaline phosphatase (up to twice normal) and falling albumin levels. The sedimentation rate and serum immunoglobulin G (IgG) levels are often much raised.

There is a statistical predominance in these patients of the histocompatibility antigen HL-A8 and, less certainly, of other antigens.

### TREATMENT

Corticosteroids rapidly improve the well-being and liver blood tests of patients with autoimmune chronic hepatitis. The survival rate is improved, particularly for younger patients with more florid disease who were likely to die in less than five years. Many patients, however, relapse, that is their liver function tests deteriorate again once corticosteroids are stopped. Even when the patient is in remission with near-normal liver blood tests and histological appearances of the liver biopsy specimen, delayed relapse can occur.

The initial dose of corticosteroids to control the inflammation in the liver is 30–40 mg prednisolone daily, reducing slowly after 2–4 weeks to a maintenance dose of 7.5–15 mg daily. If the dose of steroids to maintain remission is too high and causes side-effects such as obesity, diabetes and osteoporosis, then azathioprine 1–2 mg/kg body weight can be added, and the dose of corticosteroids reduced. Azathioprine, however, can cause leucopenia and partial loss of scalp hair.

The complications of cirrhosis are treated conventionally (*see* chapter 2).

### Hepatitis B virus active chronic hepatitis

Features of hepatitis B chronic hepatitis are shown in Table 8.3. A minority (10%) of carriers of the hepatitis B virus show aggressive rather than persistent hepatitis in liver biopsy specimens, and some of these progress within a few years of presentation to cirrhosis with jaundice, ascites and gastrointestinal bleeding.

# AETIOLOGY

There is probably continuing immunological attack on liver cells harbouring hepatitis B virus with progressive fibrosis starting around portal tracts. The virus can be detected in liver cells as the HB core antigen and later as the viral DNA in the liver cells nuclei by recombination techniques.

**Table 8.3**   Features of hepatitis B chronic hepatitis

Serum markers of HBV infection present
HBV in liver nuclei
Men > women
Homosexuals, drug addicts frequent
Prevalence increased in tropics
HL-antigens normal
Usually mild disease
No response to corticosteroids

# CLINICAL FEATURES

In Europe and the United States hepatitis B virus active chronic hepatitis predominates in men, and there is a high frequency of homosexuals and drug addicts, but this is not so in patients from tropical countries where there is much more hepatitis B, chronic hepatitis and cirrhosis. Presentation is more often by chance than with jaundice, and abnormal liver blood tests are unexpectedly found, for instance, in genitourinary medicine clinics.

Serum autoantibodies and associated diseases are unusual, but there is an association with polyarteritis syndromes such as glomerulonephritis and skin rashes. There is sometimes a history of an acute hepatitis B hepatitis, and previous episodes of hepatitis due to other viruses (i.e. hepatitis A and non-A, non-B) are frequent.

Liver function tests are usually only mildly abnormal, and jaundice comes on only late in the disease.

# TREATMENT

No treatment is effective. There is insufficient evidence that corticosteroids or azathioprine are beneficial even to the jaundiced patients. Trials of the antiviral agents interferon and adenine arabinoside are in progress. They do reduce the levels of serum markers.

118 *Chapter 8*

The complications of cirrhosis, such as ascites and oedema, gastro-intestinal bleeding and hepatoma, are treated conventionally (*see* chapter 2).

## Other causes of chronic hepatitis

Occasionally chronic, rather than acute, hepatitis is caused by prolonged administration of drugs. This is described in chapter 7. Chronic hepatitis with chronic inflammatory bowel disease is described in chapter 15, chronic, destructive, non-suppurative cholangitis (primary biliary cirrhosis), Wilson's disease and $\alpha_1$-antitrypsin deficiency in chapter 10, and alcoholic liver disease in chapter 9.

## FURTHER READING

Hoofnagle J.H. (1983) Chronic type B hepatitis. *Gastroenterology* **84**, 422–4.
McFarlane I.G. (1984) Autoimmunity in liver disease. *Clinical Science* **67**, 569–78.

# Chapter 9
# Alcoholic Disease

All forms of alcoholic liver disease are less common in the UK than in almost all other European countries. In all countries at present the consumption of alcohol is steadily increasing.

## HEPATIC EFFECTS OF ALCOHOL

Alcohol has toxic effects not only on the liver but also on many other organs.

### Drug metabolism

Large *acute* doses of alcohol impair the metabolism of drugs by the liver, presumably because the massive oxidation of alcohol inside the liver cells depletes the oxidative capacity of the cells. Acute drinking is also well known to increase, sometimes dangerously, the cerebral effects of sedatives.

*Chronic* ingestion of alcohol induces many hepatic microsomal enzymes, as well as the metabolism of alcohol itself, and so the clearance of drugs from the blood by the liver is increased and larger doses of them are needed to obtain the same pharmacological effects. This is probably most important for warfarin, as its concentration in liver cells critically controls the clotting of blood.

Alcoholics are also resistant to the effects of sedatives, but this is at least partly due to increased cerebral resistance to sedation.

Chronic ingestion of small amounts (*c.* 20g/day) of alcohol increases the plasma levels of high density lipoproteins (HDL). This is beneficial, but larger doses depress the levels.

### Fatty liver

Chronic alcohol ingestion leads to the accumulation of fat within liver cells and enlargement of the liver. This is also known as *steatosis* in some other countries. It is due both to impairment of the transport of triglycerides from the liver cell into blood on their way to peripheral tissues, and to increased intrahepatic synthesis of triglycerides. Fatty liver is reversible if the alcohol intake is reduced, and it does not itself lead to cirrhosis.

120 *Chapter 9*

The patient may present with early morning nausea and retching ('dry heaves'), or mild diarrhoea, or enlargement of the liver may be detected at a routine medical examination.

The liver is clinically enlarged, but not tender. There may be the general clinical features of the alcoholic, such as alcoholic fetor, a flushed and telangiectatic face, Dupuytren's contractures, tremor etc. (*see* chapter 1).

Investigations may reveal mildly abnormal liver blood tests, with particularly raised levels of gamma glutamyl and other transferases. Indeed these enzymes are useful for screening patients who may be drinking more alcohol than they admit!

Haemolysis and hyperlipoproteinaemia (Zieve's syndrome) can occur, and the red cells are then misshapen (spur cells). Alcohol also directly impairs the function of the bone marrow, and the red cells become larger (macrocytosis). Although macrocytosis may be also due to folate or vitamin $B_{12}$ deficiencies, alcoholism alone is a more frequent cause. A mild polycythaemia is also frequent, perhaps due to the diuretic effect of alcohol reducing the plasma volume.

Hypoglycaemia can occur with heavy drinking, and epilepsy during withdrawal from alcohol. There may be a mild hyperuricaemia and hypertriglyceridaemia.

### Alcoholic hepatitis

Continued heavy drinking can cause various degrees of acute alcoholic hepatitis in which there is damage to liver cells, infiltration of the lobule with acute inflammatory cells (polymorphonuclear leucocytes), and a characteristic accumulation within liver cells of red-staining, (eosinophilic) material called Mallory's hyaline. There may also be some fibrosis extending from the portal tracts into the lobules, and a hyaline sclerosis around central veins in the middle of the lobule.

The patient may be ill, with anorexia, vomiting, jaundice, fever, confusion, delirium and tremor, spider naevi, and sometimes an amazingly large, tender liver. There is macrocytosis, a peripheral leucocytosis, and liver blood tests show greatly raised transferases, and often conjugated hyperbilirubinaemia. The alkaline phosphatase level may be elevated in those with prolonged jaundice and cholestasis.

Although most patients improve and their appetite returns on withdrawal of alcohol, many are only mildly affected, and rapidly progressive fatal liver failure with ascites, jaundice, abnormal clotting and encephalopathy can occur, all without cirrhosis being present.

There is some evidence that high doses of corticosteroids improve the clinical course of patients with florid alcoholic hepatitis, but this is not yet

*Alcoholic Disease* 121

certain. The B complex vitamins are given intravenously (Parentrovite), but seldom with any effect; folic acid and vitamin C are given orally.

Sedation is often needed (chlormethiazole 1–3 g/day or diazepam 15–40 mg/day) for several days. Epilepsy is treated with phenytoin (150–600 mg/day).

## Alcoholic cirrhosis

### AETIOLOGY

The total dose of alcohol is important, so the longer and the more the patient drinks the more likely that cirrhosis will develop. Women are more susceptible than men. The lowest dose that leads to a statistical increase of the incidence of cirrhosis is 80 g of alcohol daily in men and 40 g in women with 1 unit of alcohol equal to 10 g. For a man this equivalent is contained in a bottle of wine, one-third of a bottle of spirits or 6 pints of normal beer (Table 9.1).

**Table 9.2**  Alcohol content in beverages

| Quantity of alcohol | Beverage |
| --- | --- |
| 10 g | 1 glass sherry or wine |
| | $\frac{1}{2}$ pint beer |
| | 1 'short' |
| 70 g | 1 bottle of wine |
| 120 g | 1 bottle of sherry |
| 250 g | 1 bottle of gin |

There is no evidence that anything in beverages other than alcohol is toxic to the liver.

Acute alcoholic hepatitis is probably pre-cirrhotic, but is usually reversible if intake is greatly reduced. Many patients with alcoholic cirrhosis, however, have had no previous episodes of acute alcoholic hepatitis.

There is no evidence that previous viral hepatitis predisposes to alcoholic cirrhosis, but a chronic hepatitis due to persistence of hepatitic B may increase susceptibility to alcohol. There may be an abnormal distribution of histocompatibility antigens in patients with alcoholic cirrhosis, suggesting

122 *Chapter 9*

some genetic predisposition, but this is debated.

The prevalence of alcoholic cirrhosis is increasing, particularly among women.

## CLINICAL FEATURES

The patient with alcoholic cirrhosis presents with the clinical features of cirrhosis described in chapter 10, but spider naevi and facial telangiectases are florid, and there may be parotid enlargement, cold sweating hands and feet, a peripheral neuropathy, dementia and muscle wasting. There could be a past history of episodes of hospital admissions for delirium tremens or jaundice.

Macrocytosis with or without anaemia may be present. Liver function tests usually reveal a moderately raised alkaline phosphatase level (2–3 times increased), and markedly elevated transferases. Jaundice, unless during an episode of hepatitis, is a late feature.

The liver may be large, due to fat, oedema and inflammation, or may have shrunk to the small liver characteristic of museum pots (Laennec's cirrhosis). It is micronodular (nodules < 5 mm diameter), and the histological appearances reveal a chronic hepatitis with portal and peripheral inflammation. There is excess iron deposited in liver cells, but less than in haemochromatosis.

## TREATMENT

The only treatment is abstinence! Some of the features of alcoholism will regress, and although cirrhosis is irreversible, survival is improved by stopping drinking. In general a diet without any alcohol is easier to maintain than one with a little!

A better diet, and a short course of the vitamin B complex, folic acid and vitamin C are given.

The complications of cirrhosis such as ascites, encephalopathy and bleeding varices are treated as in chapter 2.

### Hepatitic porphyria

Porphyria cutanea tarda, that is photosensitive skin porphyria coming on late in life, is usually found in alcoholics with cirrhosis (*see* chapter 13).

# Alcoholic Disease

## Hepatoma

There is an increased frequency of primary hepatocellular carcinomata (hepatoma) in patients with alcoholic cirrhosis (*see* chapter 11). In these patients it is a frequent cause of death.

## EXTRAHEPATIC EFFECTS OF ALCOHOL

In the alcoholic with liver disease, systems other than the liver are often as badly affected (Table 9.2).

**Table 9.2**　Effects of alcohol on non-hepatic organs

| System | Effect |
| --- | --- |
| Brain | Intoxication |
| | Epilepsy |
| | Hypoglycaemia |
| | Delirium tremens |
| | Wernicke's encephalopathy |
| | Korsakoff's psychosis |
| | Cerebellar damage |
| | Dementia |
| Nerves | Peripheral neuropathy |
| Muscles | Myopathy |
| Heart | Cardiomyopathy |
| Testes | Atrophy |
| Pancreas | Acute and chronic pancreatitis |
| Joints | Gout |
| Bone | Necrosis of femoral head |
| | Osteoporosis |
| Metabolism | Obesity |

## Neuropsychiatric complications of alcohol

### ACUTE INTOXICATION

The features of acute alcoholic intoxication are familiar, but may include delusions and hallucinations, and nystagmus. Blackouts can occur, with periods of amnesia.

# TRAUMA

Trauma is common, from bruises due to falls, to multiple rib fractures and subdural haematomata.

# EPILEPSY

Grand mal fits may follow 12–24 hours after stopping heavy alcohol intake. Focal fits, that is epilepsy starting at a given anatomical site, suggest another cause, such as cerebral trauma to which alcoholics are prone.

# HYPOGLYCAEMIA

Hypoglycaemia is unusual but important to exclude, and follows heavy drinking. It too can cause fits.

# DELIRIUM TREMENS

This dangerous state of hyperactivity has a mortality of up to 10%. Apart from the well-known frightening hallucinations, there is fever, sweating, tremor, agitation, tachycardia, dehydration and hyponatraemia.

Treatment is with sedatives (especially chlormethiazole), intravenous electrolytes and B vitamins.

# WERNICKE'S ENCEPHALOPATHY

Wernicke's encephalopathy is due to thiamine (vitamin $B_1$) deficiency. It includes ocular abnormalities, namely nystagmus and paralysis of eye movements, confusion, ataxia and peripheral neuropathy. Some cases do not respond to thiamine treatment. Haemorrhages are characteristically found *post mortem* in the pons.

# KORSAKOFF'S PSYCHOSIS

Korsakoff's psychosis is seldom reversible. There is severe loss of short-term memory, such as recalling lunch or where things were put down in a room. There is better preservation of past memories and of immediate recall, such as memorising numbers. Confabulation, or the fabrication of false stories and events, can be striking but only develops in some.

## CEREBELLAR AND CEREBRAL DEGENERATION

Irreversible damage to the cerebellum causes severe ataxia of the trunk and legs. Damage to the cortex causes dementia, namely irreversible global impairment of memory and intellect.

## PERIPHERAL NEUROPATHY AND MYOPATHY

There may be a peripheral burning feeling of the feet, and weakness with muscle tenderness. A subclinical autonomic and sensory neuropathy is frequent, and contributes to the lack of peripheral hair, cold, sweating hands and feet and impotence.

### Other complications

The heart (cardiomyopathy), testes (atrophy) and pancreas (acute and chronic pancreatitis) are all often effected by chronic abuse of alcohol. Obesity is frequent.

## SOCIALLY

The patient with alcoholic tissue damage frequently has a history of failure, lost jobs, accidents, depression, separation or divorce, crime, and addiction to other drugs. Doctors are not immune!

## FURTHER READING

Editorial (1983) Blood and alcohol. *Lancet* **1**, 397.
Editorial (1983) Immunological abnormalities in alcoholic liver disease. *Lancet* **2**, 605–6.
Pearce J.M.S. (1977) Neurological aspects of alcoholism. *British Journal of Hospital Medicine* August, 132–42.
Petersson B., Krantz P., Kristensson H., Trell E. & Sternby N.H. (1982) Alcohol-related death: A major contributor to mortality in urban middle-aged men. *Lancet* **2**, 1088–90.
Rail D.L. & Swash M. (1982) The neuropsychiatric complications of alcoholism. *Hospital Update* **8**, 463–71.
Rix K.J.B. (1978) Alcohol withdrawal states. *Hospital Update* **4**, 403–7.
Sherlock S. (1984) Nutrition and the alcoholic. *Lancet* **1**, 436–40.

# Chapter 10
# Cirrhosis

René Laennec used the word *cirrhosis* to describe the yellowish colour *post mortem* of the cirrhotic liver. Today it is defined pathologically as a combination of past and present necrosis of liver cells, inflammation, that is infiltration by inflammatory cells, fibrosis in response to the necrosis, and regeneration of liver cells into rounded nodules. Strictly these four changes must be present in the whole liver, as there are similar, rare non-cirrhotic conditions affecting only parts of the liver.

The gross appearance of the liver is often described as macronodular, micronodular or mixed, depending upon the size of the regeneration nodules. *Micronodular cirrhosis* (previously called Laennec's or portal cirrhosis, or hobnail liver) typically occurs in the alcoholic, the nodules being 1–5 mm in size, while *macronodular cirrhosis* with larger nodules is typical of biliary cirrhosis. In many livers, however, a range of nodule sizes is present, and so on the whole these descriptive terms are not useful.

Fibrosis of the liver without cell damage and/or regeneration nodules is less common in this country, but occurs, for instance, in schistosomiasis (*see* chapter 6).

## PATHOPHYSIOLOGY

The pathological changes in the liver produce two general effects. Firstly, there is liver cell failure (*see* chapter 2). There is failure of the liver cells to remove endogenous and exogenous toxins properly from the blood and to metabolise them, failure to synthesize necessary proteins etc., and failure to secrete normal bile. Liver cell failure is due to a combination of loss of normal liver cells, and to by-passing of blood within the liver past the cells, so-called intrahepatic shunting (compare pulmonary shunting in chronic lung disease). Thus, some of the blood passing through the liver is not exposed to the sinusoidal surface of cells.

Secondly, the fibrosis and nodules distort the intrahepatic architecture and increase resistance to intrahepatic blood flow and thus cause portal hypertension (*see* chapter 2). This diverts blood both past the liver, i.e. extrahepatic shunting, and also through the liver past the hepatic lobules, i.e. intrahepatic shunting, as mentioned above.

## CLINICAL FEATURES

The signs and symptoms of cirrhosis are discussed in chapter 1. The symptoms with which a patient with cirrhosis may present to the doctor are listed here:

Lethargy, weakness
Weight loss, anorexia
Ankle swelling (oedema)
Abdominal swelling (ascites)
Nausea, vomiting
Haematemesis and melaena
Failing memory, irritability, drowsiness (encephalopathy)
Jaundice, bruising

They are varied and include symptoms of associated diseases, such as alcoholism.

Common physical signs of cirrhosis include:

Obesity, wasting of limbs
Telangiectases of face, spider naevi
Bruising
Palmar erythema
White nails
Dupuytren's contracture
Clubbing
Fetor and flap
Large or small liver
Splenomegaly
Ankle oedema and ascites
Testicular atrophy; gynaecomastia

Some patients may have several signs, but many only have one or two.

**Note.** Jaundice is often *not* present. The liver can be large, normal or small. Dupuytren's contractures of the hands are a feature of alcoholism. Spider naevi develop in active cirrhosis due to alcohol or autoimmune chronic hepatitis. Itching and later xanthomata are characteristic of primary biliary cirrhosis. Clubbing of the fingers and toes and enlargement of the parotid glands are frequently searched for, but are rare.

Cirrhosis is often asymptomatic and is then found *post mortem* or at surgery.

128 *Chapter 10*

## BLOOD TESTS

The abnormalities of liver blood (function) tests in patients with cirrhosis differ. They may vary from normal to grossly abnormal. The bilirubin level is often raised in actively drinking alcoholics, in untreated autoimmune chronic hepatitis, and in primary or secondary biliary cirrhosis, in which jaundice commences early in the disease.

The alkaline phosphatase level is usually only mildly elevated (e.g. < twice normal), but in the evolution of cirrhosis is the first of the routine blood tests to become normal. It is characteristically more and earlier elevated in biliary cirrhosis.

Transferases (transaminases) are elevated when there is current active inflammation and damage to liver cells. Thus, high levels occur in the alcoholic when drinking is heavy and in autoimmune chronic hepatitis.

Serum albumin levels and the prothrombin time become abnormal when cirrhosis is advanced enough to reduce the synthesis of blood proteins by liver cells. A prolonged prothrombin time after the administration of parenteral vitamin K indicates severe liver disease (*see* chapter 3).

Serum immunoglobulins are often raised, in particular IgM in primary biliary cirrhosis and IgG in autoimmune chronic hepatitis, but these changes are not diagnostic.

## OTHER INVESTIGATIONS

A liver scan will firstly show the size of the liver, and secondly may reveal a patchily impaired uptake of the colloid by the liver, giving the appearance of filling defects. This is due mainly to shunting of blood, and to increased splenic uptake of the colloid (*see* chapter 3). Ultrasound will reveal the abnormal pattern of liver tissue, the sizes of the liver and spleen, and sometimes a dilated portal vein.

An accurate diagnosis depends upon the histological examination of a needle liver biopsy specimen. The diagnosis of cirrhosis is occasionally missed even with an adequate biopsy specimen if the needle takes tissue from the middle of a nodule. The appearance of nodules of liver cells surrounded by circular fibrosis is diagnostic. In addition, the degree of inflammation in and around the portal tracts indicates whether the disease is progressing, or active. Finally, in the specimen there may be clues to the aetiology of the cirrhosis. Thus there are fat globules in the liver of the alcoholic, periportal inflammation in autoimmune chronic hepatitis, and damage to bile ducts in primary biliary cirrhosis. Special stains may reveal excess iron or copper in liver cells, hepatitis B viral antigens, or $\alpha_1$-antitrypsin.

## AETIOLOGICAL TYPES OF CIRRHOSIS (TABLE 10.1)

**Table 10.1**   Causes of cirrhosis and resulting conditions

| Cause | Condition |
|---|---|
| **Toxins** | |
| alcohol | Alcoholic cirrhosis |
| iron | Haemochromatosis |
| copper | Wilson's Disease |
| galactose | Galactosaemia |
| drugs | Methyldopa, methotrexate |
| **Infections** | |
| hepatitis B virus<br>hepatitis non-A, non-B } | Active chronic hepatitis |
| **Cholestasis** | |
| small duct damage | Primary biliary cirrhosis |
| large duct obstruction | Secondary biliary cirrhosis |
| **Venous outflow block** | |
| large veins | Budd-Chiari syndrome<br>Chronic cardiac failure |
| small veins | Veno-occlusive disease |
| **Unknown** | |
| autoimmune (?) | Cryptogenic cirrhosis<br>Active chronic hepatitis<br>$\alpha_1$-antitrypsin deficiency |

### Alcoholic cirrhosis

Alcohol is by far the most frequent cause of cirrhosis in the UK and all developed countries, and is separately discussed in chapter 9. It is increasing in frequency everywhere due to rising alcohol consumption.

### Hepatitis B chronic hepatitis

If the hepatitis B virus persists in the liver for more than 6 months it can cause chronic hepatitis and eventually cirrhosis (*see* chapter 8). The incidence in males predominates. The cirrhosis is usually clinically and histologically

130    *Chapter 10*

inactive. Liver function tests are usually mildly abnormal; chiefly there are elevated transferase levels. The prognosis is often good, but a few patients deteriorate rapidly with cirrhosis and jaundice.

## Autoimmune chronic hepatitis

Autoimmune chronic hepatitis predominantly occurs in women and without treatment with corticosteroids progresses to cirrhosis, sometimes rapidly (*see* chapter 8). Other autoimmune diseases coexist and immunological antibodies are often found in the blood.

## Cryptogenic cirrhosis

Adult cirrhosis of unknown origin is termed cryptogenic cirrhosis, but it is probably autoimmune in origin. Its incidence in women predominates. There is little histological inflammation in the liver.

## Primary biliary cirrhosis (PBC)

Strictly primary biliary cirrhosis should be called chronic, destructive, non-suppurative cholangitis because the initial lesion is autoimmune damage to bile ducts, and cirrhosis only develops slowly. However, the simpler, less accurate name has persisted.

## HISTOLOGY

The histology of the liver is divided into three stages, although the first two stages may have been completed and cirrhosis be already present when the disease is first diagnosed.

### *State 1*

Medium-sized bile ducts in the portal tracts are surrounded by dense collections of lymphocytes and histiocytes in the form of poorly defined granulomata. The ducts are often obviously being damaged, and later they disappear.

### *Stage 2*

The number of medium-sized bile ducts are now reduced in number, but the smaller ducts proliferate, rather similarly to extrahepatic cholestasis. Chronic inflammatory cells breach the limiting plate of the portal tract into

# Cirrhosis

the periportal area of the lobule, i.e. there is chronic aggressive hepatitis.

### Stage 3

There is less inflammation but fibrosis extends into the lobule. Bile ducts are reduced or absent from many portal tracts.

### Stage 4

Cirrhosis is now present, with regeneration nodules that are often large (macronodular).

## AETIOLOGY

Primary biliary cirrhosis is probably an autoimmune disease, involving attack by immunological cells on the bile ducts, loss of ducts and, therefore, progressive intrahepatic cholestasis and eventual biliary cirrhosis.

## CLINICAL FEATURES

Women are affected nine times more than men. The typical history is of a woman, aged 40–60, who presents with progressive itching, worse at night. Xanthelasma and generalised pigmentation of the skin are followed by slowly progressive cholestatic jaundice, with dark urine, and pale stools and steatorrhoea. Lethargy increases, the liver and spleen enlarge, and clubbing may develop. Ascites, gastrointestinal bleeding from varices, widespread xanthomata and liver failure may precede death, which usually occurs 2–8 years after presentation. Some cases are, however, more benign.

Associated autoimmune diseases include an arthritis, fibrosing alveolitis of the lung, myxoedema and the sicca syndrome (dry eyes and mouth). A similar, milder liver disease occurs in a few patients with scleroderma and sarcoidosis.

## INVESTIGATIONS

Liver blood (function) tests reveal a markedly raised level of alkaline phosphatase (2–10 times normal). Later there is increasing bilirubin and falling albumin levels and eventually abnormal coagulation. The aminotransferases are only mildly raised. A mild normocytic anaemia develops. The sedimentation rate is high and immunoglobulin M levels are often raised. A high titre of seurm antimitochondrial antibody is characteristic in almost all patients, and it is also frequently detected in relatives of the

132          *Chapter 10*

patients. Smooth muscle antibody is less frequent (50%) and rheumatoid factor and antinuclear factor are found in a minority (20%).

## TREATMENT

There is no effective treatment, although some recent trials of penicillamine have reported improvement of liver blood tests, at the cost of a high frequency of major side-effects (leucopenia, skin damage). Transplantation of the liver has been tried.

Symptomatically, the itching is treated with oral cholestyramine 4 g 1–4 times daily with meals, anabolic steroids, and occasionally plasmapheresis, steatorrhea and diarrhoea are treated with a low fat diet and codeine phosphate (15–90 mg/daily). Vitamin D is given either orally, 1000 units daily, or intramuscularly, 50–150 000 units monthly, and parenteral vitamin K and A as needed. Fluid retention and gastrointestinal bleeding are treated routinely (*see* chapter 2).

The management of this slowly progressive and essentially untreatable disease over a period of years is difficult for patient and physician.

### Secondary biliary cirrhosis

This is the sequel to chronic obstruction of the extrahepatic or intrahepatic biliary tract, but only after several years. In adults the usual cause is a benign stricture of the common bile duct following difficult biliary surgery, or after a biliary-intestinal surgical bypass at the site of anastomosis of the jejunum to the upper bile duct (*see* chapter 17).

In children congenital atresia of the extrahepatic bile ducts, or the even more rare atresia of intrahepatic ducts, are eventually followed by biliary cirrhosis (*see* chapter 18).

The patient is jaundiced for many years and will often have attacks of bacterial cholangitis (*see* chapter 16). The liver is greatly enlarged, and in *post mortem* is green with large regeneration nodules (macronodular).

Treatment is surgical, if this is possible. Otherwise it is symptomatic, as for primary biliary cirrhosis.

### Haemochromatosis

Tissue damage occurs in the condition known as *haemochromatosis* due to overload of iron in the cells of various organs. Iron overload without tissue damage, and particularly without liver damage, is called *haemosiderosis*.

There are two types of haemochromatosis, namely *primary* or idiopathic, due to an inborn error of intestinal iron absorption, and *secondary*, due to

# Cirrhosis

the prolonged ingestion or intravenous administration of iron over many years. Both are uncommon.

## AETIOLOGY

In *primary haemochromatosis* the normal daily intestinal absorption of less than 10% of the normal intake of iron, i.e. 1 mg, is increased and is inappropriately high for the body stores. Normally the intestinal absorption of iron increases when the stores of iron are depleted, as after haemorrhage, and decreases when the stores are full. For an unknown reason, however, this does not correct itself in primary haemochromatosis until late in the disease. Since there is no means of excreting iron from the body, the excess slowly accumulates over many years. So the normal body stores of about 4 g of iron increases 5–10 fold, and the disease then becomes apparent.

There is an increased incidence of the disease in relatives but most cases are sporadic, that is without any familial prevalence. The condition may perhaps be inherited as an incompletely penetrating dominant characteristic, for heterozygous relatives can be shown to be mildly affected.

*Secondary haemochromatosis* usually follows repeated blood transfusions for chronic haemolytic anaemia, such as thalassaemia major. The iron in the blood cannot be excreted and after many years eventually causes tissue damage. In South Africa a heavy intake of dietary iron in the Bantu contributes to some cases of haemochromatosis.

## CLINICAL FEATURES

Primary haemochromatosis is uncommon. It predominates in males, since until the menopause or after hysterectomy or ovariectomy, menstrual blood, and therefore iron, loss protects women. The iron is particularly laid down in the liver, pancreas, skin, heart, testes and pituitary, and each organ contributes to the clinical features.

The disease normally presents in a middle-aged man with weight loss, lethargy, loss of libido and diabetes. Generalised pigmentation of the skin is noticed more by the physician than the patient. It is due to melanin accumulation in the skin, although iron does also accumulate there. It is typically greyish-brown, but often resembles normal sun tan.

The liver is enlarged, and often painful. Liver failure, jaundice and ascites are unusual as the progression to cirrhosis is slow. Diabetes develops in two-thirds, presumably due to pancreatic damage, but exocrine pancreas (enzyme) function is preserved and there is no steatorrhoea. Insulin may be needed. Testicular and pituitary function are impaired, causing testicular atrophy, impotence and infertility.

134 *Chapter 10*

A progressive congestive cardiomyopathy and chondrocalcinosis, which is arthritis associated with calcification of joint cartilages in the knee and hips, develops in a few.

Death is from hepatoma, liver failure, diabetes or cardiac failure.

### INVESTIGATIONS

The serum iron level (normal 10–30 mmol/litre; 60–160 g/dl) is raised (to > 40 mmol/litre) and there is almost complete saturation of the serum iron transport protein, transferrin. So the total iron binding capacity of the serum is normal, but the unsaturated fraction (normal *c.* 70%) is less than 10%.

The serum ferritin level is raised and is the best screening test for haemochromatosis. Ferritin is a tissue storage iron protein with a small amount in blood, and the level of the circulating fraction is proportional to body stores.

The amount of iron excreted in the urine after administration of iron chelating compounds (desferrioxamine or diethylene-triamine penta-acetic acid) is correlated with iron stores, but these tests have given way to serum ferritin levels and measurement of liver iron.

Liver blood (function) tests are only mildly abnormal, chiefly with slight elevation of the alkaline phosphatase level. A liver biopsy specimen reveals initially periportal fibrosis that extends until cirrhosis develops. Iron deposition is seen as a brown pigment that stains bright blue with Perl's prussian blue (ferrocyanide) stain in the parenchymal and Kupffer's cells. The degree of staining can be crudely graded and is proportional to the size of body stores. The amount of iron in the biopsy can also be measured by atomic absorption spectrophotometry.

### DIAGNOSIS

The chief problem is distinguishing haemochromatosis from alcoholic cirrhosis. Thus diabetes is frequent in all forms of cirrhosis, and stores of iron are often increased in the alcoholic liver. The elevation of serum ferritin levels and the amount of hepatic iron are much greater in haemochromatosis.

Iron overload also contributes to the cutaneous porphyria of the alcoholic (*see* chapter 13).

Secondary haemochromatosis is similarly looked for in multiply transfused patients.

## TREATMENT

Repeated venesection is the best treatment for primary haemochromatosis, since 1 l of blood contains 0.5 g of iron. Weekly or twice weekly 500 ml is removed until after several months the haemoglobin and serum iron and ferritin levels begin to fall. Further courses of venesection will be needed later. If the alcoholic is venesected, anaemia and iron depletion will occur more rapidly.

General health is increased, liver function and diabetes improve, pigmentation decreases and survival is lengthened.

Oral chelating agents such as ferrioxamine excrete iron in the urine, but are much less effective than venesection. Subcutaneous infusions of ferrioxamine are more effective in preventing secondary haemochromatosis, for which venesections are clearly inappropriate, but this is expensive.

Relatives, male and female, of patients with primary haemochromatosis should be screened for the incipient disease since treatment needs to be started before tissue damage occurs. Liver blood tests and serum iron and ferritin are measured, and if abnormal a liver biopsy is carried out.

### Wilson's disease

*Hepatolenticular degeneration* is another name for Wilson's disease.

## AETIOLOGY

Wilson's disease is a very rare disorder of copper metabolism, in which copper is not adequately excreted into bile and slowly accumulates in the body. It is recessively inherited.

## CLINICAL FEATURES

The intracellular copper damages the brain, particularly the basal ganglia. Damage to this causes abnormal movements and speech and rigidity, and damage to the cortex causes progressive impairment of intellect. In the liver, cirrhosis occurs usually by age 10–20 years. In the eye, copper is laid down on the posterior surface of the peripheral cornea as a ring of brownish pigment, the Kayer-Fleisher ring. It can often be seen with the naked eye, but better with the ophthalmologist's slit-lamp. In the kidney, tubular function is disturbed.

The disease usually presents in childhood either with the neurological changes or cirrhosis separately, or with both. The liver disease may present acutely with jaundice and haemolysis, or with florid active chronic hepatitis,

136 *Chapter 10*

or with portal hypertension and bleeding. The signs of liver disease may be slight, and so it should *always* be thought of in children and young adults with liver disease, particularly if there are any neurological symptoms or haemolysis.

## INVESTIGATIONS

The serum-copper containing protein caeruloplasmin is markedly reduced, and therefore the serum copper level. Urinary copper excretion is much increased, and, probably the most specifically for this disease, the liver copper concentration is increased. This may be measured in liver biopsy specimens by atomic absorption spectrophotometry, or rather unreliably by special staining of the sections. More complex studies can also be carried out with radioactive copper-67.

The eyes are examined with the slit-lamp for the rings.

## TREATMENT

Treatment is with oral penicillamine, which chelates the copper and removes it into the urine, 1–2 g daily for 1–2 years. Improvement of the clinical features is slow, and although the cirrhosis is irreversible it can be stabilised. The drug has many side-effects including skin rashes, renal damage and leucopenia, so treatment has to be carefully monitored.

Siblings must be carefully screened for the disease so that their treatment can be started before irreversible tissue damage. But tragically this is often too late by the time the disease is recognised in a family.

### Drug-induced cirrhosis

Experimental cirrhosis can be produced in animals by the chronic administration of hepatotoxins such as carbon tetrachloride, but in man drug-induced cirrhosis is rare (*see* chapter 7).

Note that acute liver damage from drugs is not followed by cirrhosis.

### *Methotrexate*

Long-standing treatment with methotrexate for psoriasis can cause cirrhosis, but many of the patients also drink much alcohol!

## Cirrhosis

### Methyldopa

An active chronic hepatitis (*see* chapter 8) and cirrhosis can develop during treatment with methyldopa, and may not be reversible.

### Oxyphenisation

Active chronic hepatitis and cirrhosis was caused by oxyphenisation in patients mainly in Australia and the United States, where it was a component of a widely used laxative.

### Alpha$_1$-antitrypsin deficiency

Severe deficiency of a serum protein, $\alpha_1$-antitrypsin, is associated with jaundice and hepatitis in neonates, with active chronic hepatitis and cirrhosis in childhood or later, and with primary emphysema of the lung in adults. Deficiency of the protein in serum is detected by electrophoresis. Histologically there are PAS (positive staining globules) in the liver cells, in which this glycoprotein is synthesised and is normally secreted into blood.

The condition is caused by homozygous inheritance of two dominant alleles. Heterozygotes have reduced serum levels but are otherwise normal.

There is no specific treatment, although corticosteroids are often given.

### Cardiac cirrhosis

Prolonged elevation of the pressure in the right atrium and therefore in the hepatic veins eventually leads to centrilobular hepatic fibrosis and cirrhosis. Cardiac cirrhosis is rare, because cardiac diseases such as constrictive pericarditis and tricuspid regurgitation are now less common in the UK and are treated surgically (*see* chapter 12).

Cirrhosis can also follow the chronic Budd-Chiari syndrome, which is obstruction of the large hepatic veins (*see* chapter 12).

## DISEASES THAT DO NOT CAUSE CIRRHOSIS

### Malnutrition

Malnutrition can cause a large fatty liver, but does not cause cirrhosis. In parts of India an unusual active cirrhosis occurs in childhood, and may be due to ingestion of an unidentified toxin. In Africa the high incidence of cirrhosis has been related to contamination of food with aflatoxin and to hepatitis B, and is not due to malnutrition.

138                                   *Chapter 10*

## Schistosomiasis

Schistosomiasis causes fibrosis of the liver and portal hypertension, but not
a true cirrhosis (*see* chapter 6).

## Congenital hepatic fibrosis

Congenital hepatic fibrosis is a rare, inherited disorder of the liver in which
there is a progressive fibrosis of the liver, but little inflammation and there
is not a true cirrhosis with nodules. It is associated with congenital lesions
of the biliary tract (*see* chapter 18), and with cysts of the liver and kidney.
There is an enlarged liver, but liver function is in general well preserved.

## FURTHER READING

Bomford A. (1979) Haemochromatosis. *Journal of the Royal Society of Medicine*
**72**, 311–4.

Dobyns W.B., Goldstein N.P. & Gordon H. (1979) Clinical spectrum of Wilson's
disease. *Mayo Clinic Proceedings* **54**, 35–42.

Editorial (1981) Alpha$_1$-antitrypsin deficiency and liver disease. *British Medical Journal* **283**, 807–8.

Gollan J.L. (1983) Diagnosis of hemochromatosis. *Gastroenterology* **84**, 418–21.

Parkes D. (1984) Wilson's disease. *British Medical Journal* **288**, 1180–1.

Powell L.W. & Halliday J.W. (1978) The detection of early hemochromatosis. *Digestive Diseases and Sciences* **23**, 377–8.

Slovis T.L., Dubois R.S., Rodgerson D.O. & Silverman A. (1971) The varied
manifestations of Wilson's disease. *Journal of Paediatrics* **78**, 578–84.

Walshe J.M. (1970) Wilson's disease: its diagnosis and management. *British Journal of Hospital Medicine* July, 91–8.

# Chapter 11
# Tumours

Tumours of the liver are either primary, that is arising from cells within the liver, or secondary, that is metastases (secondaries) to the liver from distant primary tumours.

## PRIMARY TUMOURS

### Haemangioma

#### BENIGN

Cutaneous haemangiomata or tumours of blood vessels are associated with similar benign vascular tumours of the liver. Small haemangiomata are not uncommonly found in the liver *post mortem*, but larger tumours, either *cavernous*, made up of dilated larger blood vessels, or *capillary*, consisting of proliferated small vessels, are rare.

In infancy they may present with cardiac failure and a large pulsating liver due to the large vascular shunt within it, or later present incidentally with an enlarged liver, bruit and filling defect on the liver scan or ultrasound. They may dramatically rupture spontaneously or after inadvertent needle biopsy. A plain X-ray sometimes reveals calcification within them. Thrombocytopenia can occur due to deposition of platelets within the abnormal vessels.

Treatment is usually only indicated in infancy to reduce the shunt. Corticosteroids or radiotherapy may help, but ligation of the hepatic artery or its embolisation via a percutaneous catheter are more effective. Later these tumours involute spontaneously.

#### MALIGNANT

Malignant vascular tumours are rare. They may develop many years after exposure to the obsolete radioactive X-ray contrast medium Thorotrast, which contained thorium dioxide, or after industrial exposure to vinyl chloride.

140                              *Chapter 11*

## Hepatoma

A hepatoma is a tumour of parenchymal liver cells.

## ADENOMA

Small benign adenomata, namely local overgrowth of parenchymal liver cells, are not uncommon, but larger ones are rare. They are more frequent in women taking the contraceptive pill.

## HEPATOCELLULAR CARCINOMA

Hepatocellular carcinoma is uncommon in the UK, but up to 30 times more frequent in tropical countries where it is associated with persistent carriage of the hepatitis B virus (HBV) in liver cells, and possibly with ingestion of fungal toxins. In the UK 15% occur in HBV positive patients, but most in patients with alcoholic cirrhosis (*see* chapter 9), or, much less frequently, haemochromatosis (*see* chapter 10). Hence males predominate. In the region of 20% of cases arise in normal livers.

The patient, who is often therefore known to have cirrhosis, presents with general clinical deterioration, an enlarging liver, over which occcasionally a peritoneal rub or bruit is heard, weight loss, right hypochondrial pain, ascites, or jaundice. Particularly in the Far East the carcinoma can dramatically rupture and bleed into the peritoneum, or oesophageal varices may bleed. Metabolic effects — hypercalcaemia, hypoglycaemia, polycythaemia — are occasionally seen. The hepatic veins or inferior vena cava can be invaded and cause the Budd-Chiari syndrome (*see* chapter 12). Metastasis to lung and bone is late.

The serum levels of alkaline phosphatase and later bilirubin rise. Serum $\alpha$-fetoprotein (AFP), which after infancy is normally present only in low concentrations (*see* chapter 3), is often increased. If this is more than 10 mg/ml, hepatoma is likely. About half of patients in the UK presenting with hepatomata have raised levels, but there is a greater percentage in Africa with raised levels. The ascitic fluid may be blood-stained.

A liver scan may reveal one or more filling defects, and ultrasound, computed tomography or arteriography will localise the tumour. Percutaneous or laparoscopic liver biopsy is often diagnostic.

Treatment is ineffective. Curative resection is occasionally possible, and palliative hepatic artery ligation or embolisation can reduce pain, but these are safe only if there is not cirrhosis. Radiotherapy is ineffective. The cytotoxic drug doxorubicin is being tried. Transplantation of the liver has been tried, but delayed distant metatases are frequent.

# Tumours

141

It is hoped that world-wide vaccination against HBV will reduce the incidence of this tumour, especially in countries where it is common.

## Cholangiocarcinoma

A malignant tumour of the small intrahepatic bile ducts, cholangiocarcinoma, is rare in the UK although it is frequent in the Far East where it is associated with infection of the liver with the Chinese liver fluke, *Clonorchis* (*see* chapter 6).

The clinical features are those of hepatocellular carcinoma.

Carcinomata of the larger intrahepatic and extrahepatic bile ducts are described in chapter 17.

## SECONDARY TUMOURS

It is not surprising that the largest organ in the body with one-third of the cardiac output receives many metastases from other organs, particularly from the gastrointestinal tract via the portal vein, namely the stomach, pancreas and large bowel, but also from lung, breast, kidney, and skin and eye melanomata.

Malignant lymphoid tumours also frequently involve the liver and spleen. Carcinoma of the gallbladder (*see* chapter 17) directly invades the liver. Lymph glands in the porta hepatitis may be enlarged with deposits from the stomach, pancreas and colon.

Hepatic metastases are found *post mortem* in about half the patients dying from the tumours listed previously, but they are less often detected in life. They are usually multiple rather than isolated, and may present before or after the primary tumour is obvious. Like primary hepatomata they cause a dragging right hypochondrial and epigastric ache, or peritoneal pain worse on inspiration, and jaundice or ascites may develop. The liver may become grossly enlarged, pushing up the right diaphragm and impairing breathing.

## INVESTIGATIONS

Liver blood (function) tests initially show an elevated serum alkaline phosphatase level and later bilirubin. Transferases (transaminases) are seldom much elevated. Serum albumin falls as the disease progresses, and the prothrombin time may become prolonged if cholestasis is prolonged, but it responds to parenteral vitamin K (*see* chapter 3).

Like hepatomata, diagnosis is by liver scan or ultrasound, followed by percutaneous or laparoscopic needle liver biopsy. Liver biopsy may be positive even when liver function tests are normal.

142                               *Chapter 11*

## TREATMENT

Treatment is meagre. Occasionally single metatases can be surgically resected.

Percutaneous embolisation is replacing surgical ligation of the hepatic artery. The femoral artery is catheterised and then the hepatic artery. Particles of gelfoam or freeze-dried human dura are progressively injected through the catheter and the hepatic arterial blood supply gradually reduced over 15–30 minutes. The tumours are chiefly supplied by the hepatic artery, so they necrose and collapse, and pain and hepatic enlargement are often relieved for some months.

Nausea is treated with metoclopramide (10 mg) and the disabling pain with adequate analgesia.

### Carcinoid tumours

Carcinoid tumours, which usually arise in the ileum, cause their systemic effects when they metatasise to the liver, where they then secrete their metabolically active compounds directly into the hepatic veins and thence the systemic circulation. They have a better prognosis than other metatases and survival of 5–10 years is frequent.

The systemic effects of cutaneous flushing and diarrhoea can often be controlled pharmacologically with drugs such as methysergide (2 mg tds), but careful, repeated hepatic artery embolisation is often more effective. Alternatively aggressive surgical treatment by local resection or lobectomy can be worthwhile.

### FURTHER READING

Hodgson H.J.F (1983) Primary hepatocellular carcinoma. *British Journal of Hospital Medicine* March, 240–55.

Johnson P.I. (1983) Hepatocellular carcinoma. *Hospital Update* **9**, 977–99.

Terblance J. (1977) Liver tumours. *British Journal of Hospital Medicine* February, 103–14.

# Chapter 12
# Vascular Disorders

## HEPATIC VEIN OBSTRUCTION

Partial or complete obstruction to the low pressure flow of blood through the hepatic veins and diaphragmatic inferior vena cava to the right atrium severely impairs liver function. The Budd-Chiari syndrome follows obstruction of the large hepatic veins or inferior vena cava, while veno-occlusive disease affects the small hepatic veins. Both are uncommon.

Hepatic venous congestion also occurs in severe right heart failure.

### Budd-Chiari syndrome

The large hepatic veins or upper part of the inferior vena cava can be obstructed by a thrombus, especially associated with polycythaemia, paroxysmal nocturnal haemoglobinuria, or when taking the contraceptive pill, by a local tumour such as an hepatoma or adrenal or renal carcinoma, or by a congenital web inside the upper inferior vena cava.

Sudden occlusion causes acute liver failure, with abdominal pain and rapidly enlarging liver, jaundice and ascites. Slower, less complete occlusion will eventually cause cirrhosis and portal hypertension. If the cava is blocked there is severe oedema of the legs and trunk, and albuminuria due to renal damage. *Post mortem* the cut surface of the liver resembles that of a nutmeg, with red dots representing the congested centrilobular areas.

## INVESTIGATIONS

Liver blood (function) tests are progressively abnormal, with raised bilirubin, falling albumin and increasing prothrombin time. The scintiscan may suggest the diagnosis if uptake of colloid into the caudate lobe is relatively preserved, leading to a medial 'hot spot' on the scan. This occurs because the veins of this lobe drain separately into the cava, and are often spared. Histological examination of a liver biopsy specimen will reveal centrilobular sinusoidal congestion and necrosis of liver cells, and later fibrosis proceeding to cardiac cirrhosis.

Hepatic venography via a brachial or jugular percutaneous venous

144 *Chapter 12*

catheter passed through the right atrium into the hepatic veins will show the obstruction, and also a spider-like abnormal pattern of attenuated intrahepatic veins. Opacification of the vena cava may also be needed to localise the obstruction.

## TREATMENT

Treatment is poor. The ascites is treated routinely with diuretics (e.g. spironolactone). The anticoagulant warfarin is often given, probably too late for any effect. Webs can be tackled surgically.

### Veno-occlusive disease

In animals administration of alkaloids from plants of the genera *Senecio* and *Crotalaria* cause damage to the intima of the centrilobular veins. In man ingestion of traditional Bush teas prepared from these plants, particularly in the West Indies, can lead to slow obstruction of the small intrahepatic veins. Children are the main victims. The clinical picture resembles that of the Budd-Chiari syndrome.

### Venous congestion

Raised pressures in the right atrium are transmitted to the inferior vena cava and hepatic veins, for there are no intervening valves. The liver is enlarged, and when there is tricuspid regurgitation it pulsates. Histological examination of liver biopsy specimens in patients with congestive cardiac failure will reveal centrilobular congestion.

Liver blood (function) are usually only mildly abnormal, but jaundice can occur, and may be unconjugated.

Prolonged tricuspid regurgitation or constrictive pericarditis can lead to centrilobular hepatic fibrosis and eventually cardiac cirrhosis, but this is now rare (*see* chapter 10).

## PORTAL AND SPLENIC VEIN OBSTRUCTION

Obstruction of the splenic or extrahepatic portal veins lead to left-sided portal hypertension (*see* chapter 2), splenomegaly, oesophageal varices, and sometimes ascites. It is rare in the UK but commoner in developing countries. The liver is usually normal, so liver blood tests are well preserved, and hepatic encephalopathy is unusual.

Obstruction in infancy is caused by sepsis transmitted via the umbilical vein, such as during exchange blood transfusions for anaemia or jaundice,

*Vascular Disorders* 145

or parenteral feeding. This thromboses the portal vein. Sepsis probably explains the high frequency of the thrombosis in developing countries. Thrombosis can occur spontaneously in adults with polycythaemia or taking the contraceptive pill. Tumours of the liver or pancreas may also directly involve the vessels.

The diagnosis is suspected if the liver biopsy appearances are normal in a patient with varices and splenomegaly. A percutaneous splenic venogram demonstrates the obstruction and the varices, while the wedged hepatic venous pressure (*see* chapter 3) is normal (presinusoidal portal hypertension; *see* chapter 2).

## TREATMENT

Treatment is by endoscopic sclerosis of oesophageal varices or by central or distal splenorenal shunt operations (*see* chapter 2).

## COLLAGEN DISEASES AND THE LIVER

In general the arteritis that underlies the collagen vascular disorders seldom affects the liver. Occasionally polyarteritis nodosa occludes large and small hepatic arteries and cause infarction of areas of the liver.

In systemic lupus erythematosus the liver is rarely involved. This condition should not be confused with autoimmune chronic (lupoid) hepatitis (*see* chapter 8).

In rheumatoid arthritis splenomegaly and a mild hepatic fibrosis may occur. This is called Felty's syndrome.

In scleroderma a condition similar to primary biliary cirrhosis (*see* chapter 10) occasionally occurs.

## FURTHER READING

Editorial (1979) The Budd-Chiari Syndrome. *British Medical Journal* **1**, 1302.

# Chapter 13
# Infiltration and Metabolic Disorders

## INFILTRATION OF THE LIVER

The liver is involved in many systemic conditions in which pathological tissue 'infiltrates' several organs. Liver function is usually well preserved even when the liver is greatly enlarged. Diagnosis is by histological examination of a needle biopsy specimen.

### Granulomata

*Granulomata* are discrete, localised collections of chronic inflammatory cells, namely histiocytes and lymphocytes, sometimes with a necrotic centre. They heal with fibrosis and scarring. In the liver they are scattered, but most are close to portal tracts, which when healing they may obstruct. Cell mediated immune reactions probably underlie them.

Their causes are legion and many are never discovered. Some causes of liver granulomata are:

> Sarcoidosis
> Tuberculosis (*chapter 6*)
> Drug hepatitis (*chapter 7*)
> Primary biliary cirrhosis (*chapter 10*)
> Lymphomata
> Brucellosis
> Q fever, mononucleosis (*chapter 5*)
> Inflammatory bowel disease (*chapter 15*)

Sarcoidosis and tuberculosis are the commonest. In tuberculosis the granulomata usually have caseating centres (*see* chapter 6).

### Sarcoidosis

Sarcoidosis is a rare granulomatous disease of unknown origin. There is frequently histological involvement of the liver, but clinical features are unusual. The granulomata are well demarcated and do not show caseation. They heal with fibrosis, which may slowly obliterate the portal tracts.

The liver and spleen enlarge. The alkaline phosphatase level rises, but jaundice is rare. Portal hypertension is chiefly presinusoidal (*see* chapter 2), due to obstruction of the intrahepatic portal veins.

Corticosteroids are often prescribed, but their efficacy is uncertain.

## Amyloidosis

Amyloid tissue is composed of immunoglobulin fragments laid down as a waxy infiltrate, often in many organs. It stains black with iodine like starch, hence its name. It also stains with Congo red, and is amorphous and pink with haemotoxylin and eosin stain. Polarising microscopy is diagnostic.

Secondary amyloidosis, unlike the primary form, involves the liver. This is the type that was previously often associated with chronic suppurative diseases, such as osteomyelitis, empyema, or tuberculosis. Now rheumatoid arthritis or inflammatory bowel disease are more likely, but usually the cause is unknown. The abnormal tissue is perireticular, being laid down around blood vessels, and in the liver infiltrates in the space of Disse between the liver cell columns and blood sinusoids. The spleen and kidney are also usually involved.

The liver and spleen are enlarged. Liver function is usually preserved, and jaundice is unusual. Liver histology is diagnostic. Proteinuria and renal failure are frequent.

There is no specific treatment.

## Lymphomata

Malignant cells of the retculoses invade the portal tracts. The portal tracts are enlarged and histologically appear dense due to the dark nuclei of the accumulated cells, which cytologically may be recognisably malignant. Granulomata are a feature of Hodgkin's disease.

The liver may be enlarged, and occasionally jaundice is a feature. This is usually from haemolysis, but occasionally it is due to the mechanical effects of the deposits or to an ill-understood intrahepatic cholestasis.

The diagnosis of a lymphoma is sometimes made from the appearances of the liver biopsy specimen, but often the biopsy has been performed to establish the cause of the jaundice in a patient known to have a lymphoma.

Treatment is by chemotherapy of the primary disease.

## Fatty liver

Since the liver is central in the balance between the breakdown and synthesis of adipose tissue, triglycerides are readily laid down in liver cells.

148 *Chapter 13*

Histologically they are seen as globular spaces in the liver cells left after fixing and these stain bright red with, for instance, Sudan III stain. The liver is enlarged and pale.

Fatty liver is sometimes called steatosis, but this implies that the condition is itself damaging, which it is not. Liver function is unaffected.

Fatty liver is seen in obesity, and in diabetics. It is an early and marked feature of alcoholism, when it may be combined with degrees of alcoholic hepatitis (*see* chapter 9). It is particularly striking in fatty liver of pregnancy (*see* chapter 14), in which the fat is microvesicular in tiny intracellular droplets.

In the rare Reye's syndrome of childhood, young children suddenly develop a large, fatty liver, liver failure and encephalopathy. The aetiology is not known.

Fat can be found in the liver of patients with severe inflammatory bowel disease. Fatty liver is also a feature after small bowel bypass operations for morbid obesity. In kwashiorkor fatty liver is a feature but regresses completely when nutrition is improved, without permanent effects.

## METABOLIC DISORDERS

Those disorders that are based upon metabolic enzyme defects in the liver frequently cause hepatomegaly and sometimes serious liver disease.

### Diabetes

In insulin-requiring type I diabetes, hepatomegaly can be marked when the diabetes is not controlled. It is chiefly due to an excess of glycogen laid down in liver cells, and partly to triglycerides. Liver blood (function) tests are mildly abnormal. It is reversed by treatment of the diabetes with insulin.

### Galatosaemia

A congenital deficiency of the enzyme galactose-1-phosphate uridyl transferase leads to the accumulation of toxic amounts of galactose-1-phosphate in liver cells, derived from hydrolysis of the disaccharide lactose in milk.

Vomiting, diarrhoea and jaundice usually start in infancy, with hepatosplenomegaly, cataracts, and mental retardation. Cirrhosis develops, and can present later in childhood.

Treatment is withdrawal of lactose, i.e. milk, from the diet.

## Glycogen storage disease

Congenital deficiencies of various enzymes of glycogen metabolism lead to different metabolic disorders, several of which involve the liver. Impairment of the breakdown of glycogen leads to varying degrees of glycogen accumulation in the liver and heart, and to hypoglycaemia.

The liver is greatly enlarged and laden with glycogen, but liver function is usually normal. The diseases present in infancy and stunt growth. Liver transplantation has been tried in a few of these children to correct the underlying enzymic defect.

## Porphyria

Porphyrins are intermediates in the synthesis of haem (Figure 13.1). In the final step iron is incorporated into protoporphyrin. Deficiency is one or more of the enzymes involved in the pathway causes some of the intermediates to accumulate and be excreted in excess of bile and urine. If they accumulate in the skin they cause photosensitive cutaneous blistering, and in the liver occasionally cause damage. They are divided into erythropoietic (e.g. congenital porphyria) and hepatic types (Tables 13.1 and 13.2).

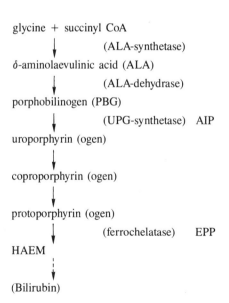

Fig. 13.1   Porphyrin pathway.

150                     *Chapter 13*

**Table 13.1**   Classification of porphyrias

| Type | Metabolic disorder |
|------|-------------------|
| Erythropoietic | Congenital porphyria |
| Hepatic | Porphyria cutanea tarda (symptomatic)<br>Acute (intermittent) porphyria<br>Variegate porphyria<br>Coproporphyria |
| Erythrohepatic | Protoporphyria |

**Table 13.2**   Sites of excess porphyrins and precursors in porphyrias

| | Urine | Stool | Red cells |
|---|-------|-------|-----------|
| Acute porphyria | Precursors —<br>ALA & PBG | Normal | Normal |
| Porphyria cutanea tarda | Uroporphyrin | Coproporphyrin | Normal |
| Erythropoietic<br>protoporphyria | Normal | Protoporphyrin | Protoporphyrin |

## ACUTE INTERMITTENT PORPHYRIN

In acute intermittent porphyria (AIP) there is a deficiency of the enzyme UPG synthetase and the porphyrin precursors porphobilinogen and aminolaevulinic acid accumulate in the liver, pass into urine, and cause neurological disorders and abdominal pain. This is a rare condition. There is no liver disease. Porphyrins are normal.

## PORPHYRIA CUTANEA TARDA

Porphyria cutanea tarda, or late onset porphyria or symptomatic porphyria, causes photosensitive blistering and scarring of the exposed face, neck and

# Infiltration and Metabolic Disorders

hands in middle age. The patient is usually male with alcoholic cirrhosis. Uroporphyrin is excreted in excess in the urine and accumulates in the liver, and coproporphyrin is excreted in the faeces. Both urine and liver biopsy specimens fluoresce in ultraviolet light due to the excess porphyrins. Examination of the liver biopsy specimen reveals cirrhosis and iron deposition. The enzyme defect is complex.

The condition responds to alcohol withdrawal and repeated venesection which removes the iron from the liver (*see* chapter 10).

## ERYTHROPOIETIC PROTOPORPHYRIN

In erythropoietic protoporphyria (EPP) or erythrohepatic porphyria, protoporphyrin accumulates in the liver, skin and red cells and initially causes a burning photosensitivity, but not blistering. The protoporphyrin may accumulate as plugs in bile canaliculi and cause cholestasis and rapid liver failure.

Gall stones containing protoporphyrin are frequent. Cholestyramine has been given to try to bind the porphyrin in the intestine and increase its excretion.

## FURTHER READING

Behrman R.E. & Vaughan V.C. (eds) (1983) *Nelson's Textbook of Paediatrics*. 12th edition. Saunders, Philadelphia.

Bloomer J.R. (1976) The hepatic porphyrias. *Gastroenterology* **71**, 689–701.

Lehmuskallio E., Hannuksela M. & Halme H. (1977) The liver in sarcoidosis. *Acta Medica Scandinavica* **202**, 289–93.

Levy M., Polliack, A., Lender M. & Eliakim M. (1974) The liver in amyloidosis. *Digestion* **10**, 40–51.

Mir-Madjlessi S.H., Farmer R.G. & Hawk W.A. (1974) Spectrum of hepatic manifestations of granulomatous hepatitis of unknown aetiology. *American Journal of Gastroenterology* **62**, 221–39.

Samson D. (1980) The porphyrias. *Hospital Update* **6**, 567–82.

Scheuer P.J. (1982) Hepatic granulomas. *British Medical Journal* **285**, 833–4.

# Chapter 14
# Pregnancy

Palmar erythema and a few spider naevi are normal in pregnancy and do not usually indicate any liver disease. They disappear after delivery.

Liver blood (function) tests are normal apart from an increase of the alkaline phosphatase level particularly in the last trimester. This is due to the isoenzyme released from the placenta, and γ-glutamyl transpeptidase levels remain normal. Sensitive tests of liver function, such as the bromsulphthalein test (*see* chapter 3), however, reveal slight impairment of bile secretion (i.e. subclinical cholestasis), and this can be reproduced by administering oestrogens to animals or humans.

### Viral hepatitis

Viral hepatitis is now less common in this country and is not any different if it occurs in pregnancy. In developing countries, however, it appears to have a high mortality when it occurs in pregnancy. It probably does not damage the fetus, nor cause malformations.

Hepatitis B in the mother can be transmitted to her baby during delivery (*see* chapter 5).

### Toxaemia

If severe, toxaemia in pregnancy causes shock-like lesions in the liver with centrilobular necrosis, but the non-hepatic features of this condition are more important.

### Fatty liver

A rare but tragic condition, fatty liver occurs late in the last trimester. Vomiting, abdominal pain, jaundice and encephalopathy rapidly develop, followed by renal failure and sometimes hypoglycaemia. Many mothers die with their fetuses. Recovery, if it occurs, is complete.

Macroscopically the liver is yellow, and histologically the liver cells are full of fat droplets. The cause is unknown, although some cases were previously associated with the administration of large intravenous doses of

# Pregnancy

tetracycline.

Treatment is that of liver failure (*see* chapter 2).

## Cholestatic jaundice

One in 2000–8000 pregnant women develop itching with or without jaundice in the third trimester or when taking the contraceptive pill if this contains oestrogen. It is thought that these women are idiosyncratically sensitive to the normal cholestatic effects of endogenous or exogenous oestrogens. It is more distressing than harmful, but it does increase the risk to the fetus.

In the first pregnancy, itching rather than jaundice is usually the main feature, but jaundice develops in later pregnancies. It rapidly remits after delivery without sequelae.

The serum bilirubin is conjugated and the urine dark, and the alkaline phosphatase level rises.

Oral cholestyramine helps the itching. Reassurance is important. Vitamin K is given intramuscularly.

## Gall stones

The incidence of gall stones is not increased in pregnancy, but until delivery radiographs cannot be used to diagnose them. Fortunately ultrasound is now available and is safe to the fetus.

High placental alkaline phosphatase levels can be confused with the elevation of the liver isoenzyme that occurs when stones cause cholestasis.

## FURTHER READING

Editorial (1983) Acute fatty liver of pregnancy. *Lancet* **1**, 339–40.
Riely C.A. (1984) Acute fatty liver of pregnancy. *Digestive Diseases and Sciences* **29**, 456–7.

# Chapter 15
# Bowel Disease

Carcinomata of the stomach and large bowel frequently metastasise to the liver (*see* chapter 11). Diarrhoea is frequent in chronic liver disease (i.e. cirrhosis), particularly if there is jaundice and cholestasis when a deficiency of bile acids in the small intestinal lumen during a meal leads to fat maldigestion and thus to steatorrhoea and diarrhoea (*see* chapter 2).

### Inflammatory bowel disease

Several different diseases of the liver and biliary tract may develop in patients with inflammatory bowel disease, both ulcerative proctocolitis and Crohn's disease. They are usually in patients with total colitis affecting the whole colon.

## FATTY LIVER

Fat droplets accumulate in liver cells in patients with chronic, severe bowel disease, particularly if they are systemically ill.

## PERICHOLANGITIS

There is chronic inflammation in the portal tracts concentrating on the bile ducts with pericholangitis. Fibrosis develops around the bile ducts, and cirrhosis can eventually follow. Jaundice may occur, but more usually there is only elevation of the level of serum alkaline phosphatase. Liver biopsy is needed for diagnosis.

There is no treatment, and colectomy does not affect it.

## SCLEROSING CHOLANGITIS

Chronic, irregular sclerosis chiefly affects the extrahepatic bile ducts, but it often extends up to the intrahepatic ducts. The aetiology is unknown, and so it is termed primary sclerosing cholangitis (*see* chapter 18). Colectomy is of no value.

## Bowel Disease

155

## BILE DUCT CARCINOMA

Carcinomata of the large bile ducts are more common than expected in patients with inflammatory bowel disease, but it is rare even in them (*see* chapter 17).

## ACTIVE CHRONIC HEPATITIS

A chronic aggressive hepatitis starting in the portal tracts may be the presenting feature of a patient with a subclinical colitis, or it may develop later during the prolonged course of colitis. Cirrhosis may follow. Conversely, more patients with chronic hepatitis than expected have autoimmune diseases such as colitis (*see* chapter 8).

It is difficult to distinguish this histologically from pericholangitis.

## FURTHER READING

Editorial (1976) An unusual cholangitis. (Sclerosing cholangitis.) *British Medical Journal* **2**, 1090–1.

Peorett A.D., Higgins G., Johnston H.H., Massarella G.R., Truelove S.C. & Wright R. (1971) The liver in Crohn's disease. *Quarterly Journal of Medicine* **40**, 187–209.

Peorett A.D., Higgins G., Johnston H.H., Massarella G.R., Truelove S.C. & Wright R. (1971) The liver in ulcerative colitis. *Quarterly Journal of Medicine* **40**, 211–38.

# Chapter 16
# Gall Stones

Gall stones are solid concretions formed in bile and found in the biliary tract, or occasionally the intestine. They are a common cause of morbidity and mortality in the developed countries. Thus in the United States 15 million people, or 12% of the adult population, have gall stones. Each year 400 000 operations are carried out for stones at a cost of 1.5 billion dollars, and 4000 patients die from the complications of stones or their surgery.

## TYPES OF GALL STONE

There are three types of gall stone: pigment, pure cholesterol and mixed.

### PIGMENT STONES

Pigment stones (10%) are black, small and crumble easily. They contain large amounts of bile pigments, including unconjugated bilirubin, and are never radio-opaque, that is they are not seen on a plain X-ray.

They are found more frequently in patients with excess haemolysis, with cirrhosis, or chronic bacterial cholangitis due to congenital and other abnormalities of the biliary tract, and in the rural population of the Far East.

Similar stones containing protoporphyrin develop in protoporphyria (*see* chapter 13).

### CHOLESTEROL STONES

Pure cholesterol stones (10%) are composed of almost pure cholesterol and are never radio-opaque.

### MIXED STONES

Mixed stones are the most frequently occurring stones (80%). They are composed of cholesterol, several calcium salts, and a small amount of pigment and protein. Their cut surface is laminated like an onion.

Ten per cent of all gall stones are radio-opaque, and they are all mixed stones.

## Gall Stones

Mixed stones are more common in women before the menopause, but become equal with men in older age groups, in the obese, and after resection or disease of the ileum. They are more frequent in Western Europe, North America and Australia than in developing countries.

## PATHOPHYSIOLOGY

A gall stone represents the gradual collection of insoluble material from bile. Once the small central nidus has precipitated or seeded from solution in bile, further material is probably then more readily laid down on it.

Pigment stones are due to water insoluble bilirubin precipitating from bile. Normally bilirubin in bile is almost all conjugated, and thus water soluble, but if it is deconjugated by the enzyme glucuronidase, which cleaves off the glucuronic acid molecules, then it will quickly precipitate. This enzyme is present in normal bile, but is also present in bacteria when there is biliary infection (i.e. cholangitis). Calcium is also probably important in decreasing the solubility of bilirubin.

Cholesterol and mixed stones are probably related to an imbalance of the amounts of cholesterol, lecithin, bile acids and calcium in bile. If there is insufficient bile acids and lecithin the micelles they form will be inadequate to keep the water insoluble cholesterol in solution, and so it starts to precipitate in layers on an initial nidus of calcium and bile pigment. This mechanism will be more likely if the liver secretes 'lithogenic' bile, that is bile from which cholesterol readily precipitates *in vitro*. Such bile may be formed because there is an insufficient pool of bile acids circulating around between liver, bile and intestine (enterohepatic circulation). This in turn arises because the synthesis of new bile acids in the liver is set at too low a level to maintain an adequate pool size of bile acids to compensate for the intestinal loss into the colon and faeces.

The reason for the female preponderance of gall stones is not known, although it may be the effect of oestrogens on bile formation. When there is disease or surgical resection of the ileum, which is where conjugated bile acids are reabsorbed in the enterohepatic circulation, the bile acid pool is reduced and hence bile is more lithogenic and stones form more frequently.

## COMPLICATIONS

Even a single stone in the biliary tract can cause one or more of various complications, depending upon whether it causes obstruction or infection of the gallbladder or common bile duct.

158    *Chapter 16*

Complications of gall stones include:

pain (colic)
jaundice (cholestasis)
acute cholecystitis
empyema of gallbladder
mucocele
chronic cholecystitis
      calcified (porcelain) gallbladder
      calcified (limey) bile
strawberry gallbladder
cholangitis
bile duct stricture
biliary cirrhosis
acute pancreatitis
gall stone ileus

## Pain

Typically gall stones cause a right hypochondrial and/or epigastric pain, sometimes radiating to the back round the right lower ribs. It can vary in intensity, with spasms or colic lasting 15–30 minutes. Colic is often thought to indicate the passage of a stone through the papilla. The pain is more constant in chronic cholecystitis and less severe. The pain of acute cholecystitis is due to inflammation extending to the peritoneum over the gallbladder. At other times gallbladder pain is presumably due to stretching of its wall, and pain from common bile duct stones may be from stretching of the duct.

Many stones, however, are painless, particularly in the elderly, and are found by chance at surgery or *post mortem*, or they present to the doctor as painless jaundice.

## Jaundice

If a stone or stones block the common hepatic or bile ducts extrahepatic cholestatic jaundice results. The stone need not be 'jammed', and indeed during cholangiography stones can be seen to roll up and down the duct and yet cause jaundice; this is perhaps because of associated infection of the bile, or because pressures within the hepatic ducts are increased. Jaundice can also occur with acute cholecystitis even when the bile ducts are free of stones, perhaps due to the inflammation extending to the adjacent common bile duct. In long-standing obstruction the dilated ducts are found to contain colourless or 'white' bile.

Typically there are also raised levels (2–5 times) of alkaline phosphatase

## Gall Stones 159

in the blood and moderate elevation of aminotransferases and gamma glutamyl transpeptidase (5–10 times elevated). The prothrombin time remains normal unless cholestasis lasts some weeks, and then it corrects with parenteral vitamin K (*see* chapter 3).

A plain X-ray may reveal air in the biliary tract if a stone has been recently passed, or calcified stones either in the gallbladder or, less commonly, in the common bile duct. Ultrasound detects gallbladder stones better than those in the bile ducts, and will also detect dilatation of the biliary tract. A CT scan will also be useful in showing dilated ducts.

Cholecystography and intravenous cholangiography are useless if the patient is jaundiced, for the contrast medium will not be excreted into bile by the liver cells. Percutaneous or retrograde cholangiography are therefore the procedures of choice for diagnosis of jaundice (*see* chapter 3).

### Acute cholecystitis

When a stone or stones causes a bacterial infection of the bile in the gallbladder and its wall acute cholecystitis occurs. The inflammation extends to the peritoneal covering and causes local peritonitis. *Escherichia coli* and *Streptococci* are the usual organisms; cholecystitis also occurs in typhoid fever.

The patient complains of right hypochondrial pain, often with vomiting, and there is local tenderness over the gallbladder, a positive Murphy's sign, local rebound tenderness and sometimes a palpable mass due to distension of the gallbladder or to omentum wrapping the inflamed organ. Fever and leucocytosis occur. Jaundice is unusual, but liver enzymes are often raised.

The episode will usually settle with antibiotic treatment and intravenous fluids. It may be followed by chronic cholecystitis, or a chronic abscess, namely an empyema of the gallbladder. If the cystic duct remains blocked the pigment etc. of the stagnant bile is absorbed and white mucus fills the gallbladder, which is a mucocele of the gallbladder.

The timing of cholescystectomy is controversial. Surgery during the acute stage is difficult, but the illness is shortened. Alternatively, after recovery an elective cholecystectomy is carried out if ultrasound or cholecystography demonstrate stones still to be present. Cholangiography or choledochoscopy (examination of the inside of the main bile ducts with a narrow fibreoptic endoscope) should always be performed during the operation.

### Chronic cholecystitis

When there are long-standing stones in the gallbladder chronic cholecystitis occurs. They set up sterile or bacterial inflammation in the wall of the

160 *Chapter 16*

gallbladder, which becomes thickened and shrunken, with loss of normal mucosa.

Chronic cholecystitis due to gall stones can cause right hypochondrial and epigastric pain and mimic true dyspepsia, but its relation to nausea, heartburn, bloating, eructation and fat intolerance is unproven. There may be local tenderness and a positive Murphy's sign. Liver function tests are normal. The only treatment of chronic cholecystitis is cholecystectomy, but it is doubtful that this should be done unless gall stones are definitely present.

Occasionally calcium is laid down in the wall of the gallbladder with chronic cholecystitis, and then it becomes radio-opaque on a plain X-ray of the abdomen (*porcelain gallbladder*). Another unusual radiological finding is '*limey bile*', when the calcium in the bile makes it milky and the whole gallbladder is radio-opaque.

### Strawberry gallbladder

The mucosa of the gallbladder has an unusual appearance when viewed macroscopically looking like the speckled surface of a ripe strawberry. This is due to deposition of lipids in the mucosa. There are no symptoms, but stones are often present.

### Ascending cholangitis

Infection of the bile ducts is usually due to intestinal bacteria, but they may reach the ducts through the bloodstream rather than 'ascending' from the duodenum.

Ascending cholangitis is always associated with partial or complete obstruction of the bile ducts, most commonly from stones, but also from benign or malignant strictures, congenital abnormalities of the ducts, or occasionally from worms (Ascaris) or the liver fluke (Clonorchis) in tropical countries (*see* chapter 6). The patient develops a swinging fever, sometimes with rigors and jaundice. This used to be called Charcot's intermittent biliary fever or Charcot's triad. There is also right hypochondrial pain and hepatic tenderness.

If the infection spreads, septicaemia, shock and renal failure can lead to death. Multiple pyogenic intrahepatic abscesses used to be frequent. Before modern antibiotics, particularly those effective against anaerobic and microaerophilic organisms, urgent surgical intervention was mandatory, but now a trial of intensive medical treatment after blood cultures have been set up is first indicated. The obstruction and abscesses (*see* chapter 6) can be seen with ultrasonography, or with percutaneous cholangiography when bile can be obtained for culture. Needling the liver, however, can precipitate

## Gall Stones

septicaemia, and antibiotics, such as amoxycillin and gentamicin must be given during and after the procedure.

### Bile duct stricture

Benign strictures are secondary to gall stones or to surgery.

### Biliary cirrhosis

Secondary biliary cirrhosis is now uncommon, but used to follow obstruction of the bile ducts for many years, or more commonly after repeated cholangitis from a stricture. It is characterised by prolonged jaundice and eventually a large, knobbly, macronodular liver. For biliary cirrhosis *see* chapter 10.

### Acute pancreatitis

Acute pancreatitis is frequently caused by the passage of a small stone through the ampulla of Vater in some way obstructing or causing reflux of bile into the pancreatic duct. Chronic pancreatitis is probably not related to gall stones.

### Gall stone ileus

Intestinal obstruction can be caused by a large gall stone that has perforated through the wall of the gallbladder and ruptured into the duodenum through this fistula, or even by one that has managed to pass through the ampulla. It is uncommon, and usually found in the elderly.

### TREATMENT

### Surgical

Surgical treatment of gall stones is traditional and therefore discussed before medical treatment. The older operations for gall stones have been replaced by cholecystectomy, or removal of the gallbladder and part of the cystic duct. Every cholecystectomy should, if it is possible, include direct cholangiography on the operating table or endoscopic choledochoscopy to look for small, missed stones; otherwise cholestatic jaundice a few days after surgery will occasionally occur.

The indications for cholecystectomy include acute cholecystitis, a previous episode of acute cholecystitis, chronic cholecystitis if stones have been diagnosed by ultrasonography or cholecystography, or carcinoma of the gallbladder.

162 *Chapter 16*

## POSTCHOLECYSTECTOMY SYNDROME

Some patients may have right hypochondrial pain some time after cholecystectomy. A few are found on percutaneous or retrograde cholangiography to have stone(s) in the common bile duct, but most of these stones have probably formed *de novo* after surgery, only a few being left at surgery (i.e. retained stones). The role of biliary spasm in this syndrome is unproven.

If there are no stones, management is difficult. Many are suffering from colonic pain.

### Medical

### PHARMACOLOGICAL DISSOLUTION

Dissolution of stones was widely attempted in the nineteenth century with oral chloroform, ether and olive oil, but apart from analgesia there was until recently no effective means of dissolving stones. It is now clear that over many months large doses of the natural dihydroxy bile acids, chenodeoxycholic and ursodeoxycholic acids, will slowly dissolve many gall stones in the gallbladder. The stones must be radiolucent, for if radio-opaque they contain too much calcium to dissolve. The gallbladder must also be functioning, that is opacify on cholecystography. Otherwise, like the contrast medium, the bile acids will not get into the gallbladder. Large stones take much longer to dissolve than small stones, and the dose has to be tailored to the body weight (*c.* 15 mg/kg). Diarrhoea can be a problem with chenodeoxycholic acid.

Unfortunately a proportion of stones recur a few months after stopping treatment, so at present this treatment is only indicated if there is a special reason for advising against surgery, such as those with young children at home, or because of age or infirmity. However, for such groups this treatment is an advance, and is a treatment specifically designed from an understanding of the physiology of bile acids. The increased concentration of the administered bile acid in bile is thought both to decrease the secretion of cholesterol into bile by the liver and slowly to dissolve the cholesterol from the stones.

### Endoscopic

It has recently become possible to perform a sphincterotomy of the ampulla of Vater through a fibreoptic duodenoscope. A diathermy wire is introduced into the bile duct, and its wall and the duodenal mucosa overlying it are slit up for 1–2 cm. The stones in the bile duct will either pass spontaneously

## Gall Stones

into the duodenum or can be withdrawn with a small wire basket introduced again through the duodenoscope. This procedure is now taking the place of the difficult second surgical operation for bile duct stones developing after cholecystectomy, and as a first procedure in the elderly.

### T-TUBE REMOVAL

The surgeon may leave a large bore T-tube in the common bile duct at the time of cholecystectomy. If a stone is then seen on the T-tube cholangiogram to have been left behind, it can be removed with a steerable catheter and basket passed along the tract of the T-tube into the bile duct under radiological control.

### FURTHER READING

Bouchier I.A.D. (1983) Gall stone dissolving agents. *British Medical Journal* **286**, 778–80.

Classen M. & Schreiber H.W. (eds) (1983) Biliary tract disorders. *Clinics in Gastroenterology* **12**, No 1.

Cotton P.B. (1984) Endoscopic management of bile duct stones. *Gut* **25**, 587–97.

Schoenfield L.J. (1977) *Diseases of the Gall Bladder and Biliary System*. Wiley, New York.

# Chapter 17
# Tumours of the Biliary Tract

Almost all primary tumours of the biliary tract arise from its mucosa and are usually adenocarcinomata. They present with jaundice due to extrahepatic obstruction of the bile flow, i.e. cholestasis. The effects of a carcinoma of the head of the pancreas and chronic pancreatitis on the biliary tract are also described here, but the former only invades the common bile duct and is not a primary tumour, and in the latter the non-malignant swollen gland presses on the duct.

### Diagnosis

*Courvoisier's law* emphasises that in a patient jaundiced from gall stones, the gallbladder is small and impalpable due to past chronic cholecystitis, while carcinomata of the pancreas invade the common bile duct and cause dilatation of the biliary tract including the gallbladder above the obstruction, so that the distended gallbladder may be palpable in the right hypochrondrium. However, because there are so many exceptions, and because a large gallbladder can be difficult to feel, this 'law' is unreliable. Otherwise diagnosis depends upon the diagnostic methods described in chapters 3 and 4.

## CARCINOMA OF THE GALLBLADDER

Carcinoma of the gallbladder is an uncommon tumour arising in the elderly in a gallbladder containing stones. It presents with a right hypochondrial pain, weight loss, or jaundice if it has invaded the main duct or metastasized to the lymph glands in the hilum of the liver.

A hard mass may be palpable in the right hypochondrium, but usually the diagnosis is unexpectedly made at surgery. The tumour has in most cases already spread directly into the liver or via lymphatics, and so curative reaction is rarely possible. Radiotherapy is of limited value.

## CARCINOMA OF THE BILE DUCTS

Carcinoma may arise in any part of the extrahepatic tree or the large intrahepatic ducts. Tumours of the small intrahepatic ducts are called cholangiocarcinomata of the liver and are described in chapter 11.

Bile duct carcinomata are usually slowly growing, mucus secreting, scirrhous adenocarcinomata that may spread along the ducts. They can be difficult to distinguish even histologically from benign fibrosis of the ducts, that is sclerosing cholangitis (*see* chapter 18).

## Clinical features

Carcinoma of the bile ducts present with cholestatic jaundice in the elderly.

## Diagnosis

Diagnosis is dependent upon radiology of the biliary tract, namely percutaneous or retrograde cholangiography, and these procedures are useful for showing the upper and lower extent of the tumour. Above the tumour the ducts may be grossly dilated, and little or no dye may pass either way through the stricture. Ultrasonography or CT scanning will detect larger tumours.

## Treatment

Treatment is by resection of this slow growing tumour, if this is possible, and anastomosis of the proximal bile duct or gallbladder above the stricture to a Roux-en-Y loop of small intestine (i.e. a cholecyst or a choledochojejunostomy). Alternatively a palliative drainage with an intestinal loop anastomosed to the hilar ducts and leaving the tumour *in situ* may be all that is possible; or at surgery a stent can be passed through the tumour and left in place, which is called internal drainage.

Recently techniques for either retrograde or transhepatic drainage without surgery have been developed. With retrograde drainage, a small looped catheter is passed up through the ampulla of Vater from the duodenum via a fibreoptic duodenoscope so that it spans the stricture. With transhepatic drainage a wire is passed percutaneously into and through the liver and down through the stricture. A short catheter stent is then run along the wire and pushed through the stricture by means of a catheter behind it. The stent is then left in place as an internal splint, and the wire and catheter removed. Clearly both techniques are only palliative, but since tumour growth is slow, jaundice can be relieved for many months.

Radiotherapy is used, but is of limited value. A recent method is to insert a wire containing radioactive iridium percutaneously or at surgery through the stricture and this gives high dose local irradiation, and then can be removed.

166 *Chapter 17*

Drainage of the dilated hepatic ducts with an indwelling percutaneous catheter in the liver and draining into a bag (external drainage) has been used, is technically easy and rapidly relieves jaundice. However, it causes too many complications.

## CARCINOMA OF THE AMPULLA

Carcinoma of the ampulla is an adenocarcinoma in or close to the papilla of Vater, and arising from the lower end of the common bile duct or the pancreatic duct, or probably also from nearby pancreatic acini. The peak age of incidence is 50–70 years.

### Clinical features

Jaundice occurs early due to obstruction of the bile duct, and therefore the tumour may present when it is still small. Steatorrhoea and/or diarrhoea is due to obstruction of the pancreatic duct and impaired secretion of exocrine enzymes. Iron deficiency anaemia or frank melaena may occur if the tumour bleeds into the duodenum. Occasionally the silver stool, the combination of black melaena and yellow steatorrhoea, is noticed. Serum amylase levels may be raised. Later the duodenum may become obstructed by the enlarging tumour and then the syndrome of pyloric stenosis develops, with vomiting and rapid weight loss.

### Diagnosis

Diagnosis can sometimes be made on a careful barium meal when there is a constant filling defect on the medial wall of the second part of the duodenum. More directly, endoscopic duodenoscopy will reveal swollen, irregular mucosa that bleeds easily in the region of the papilla, and biopsy and brush specimens can be obtained for histology and cytology. Both percutaneous and retrograde cholangiography will delineate the site of the bile duct obstruction, and a pancreatogram obtained at the same time will show dilatation of the pancreatic ducts proximal to the tumour.

### Treatment

The prognosis is poor, but better than for other pancreatic adenocarcinomata since some can be successfully resected. To do this, however, the duodenum, the head of the pancreas and the lower common bile duct must be excised and a cholecyst jejunostomy or choledochojejunostomy, gastrojejunostomy and anastomosis of the pancreatic stump to the bowel must all be carried out.

*Tumours of the Biliary Tract* 167

This is Whipple's operation. Because it carries a high morbidity and mortality, it is only justified in younger and fitter patients with no evidence of spread of the tumour obtained before or at surgery.

If age, poor health or evidence of spread preclude surgery, then palliation as for bile duct carcinomata can be considered. Radiotherapy is also sometimes tried.

## CARCINOMA OF THE PANCREAS

Adenocarcinomata rising in the acini of the head of the pancreas can cause jaundice by obstructing the common bile duct either as it passes behind the pancreas, or higher up. They occur chiefly between the ages of 50 and 70 and are more frequent in smokers.

### Clinical features

Apart from cholestatic jaundice, carcinoma of the pancreas may also cause abdominal and back pain, anorexia and weight loss, steatorrhoea and/or diarrhoea, and diabetes mellitus. Thrombophlebitis migrans, that is one or more painful, local areas of thrombophlebitis, usually in the legs, may also occur. The reason is not known. Later, obstruction of the duodenum may cause the syndrome of pyloric stenosis with vomiting. The gallbladder may be palpable. Large pancreatic carcinomata can sometimes be palpated in the epigastrium.

### Diagnosis

Serum amylase levels are sometimes raised, and hyperglycaemia and glycosuria are frequent, but not invariable.

The barium meal may reveal distortion of the medial wall of the duodenal loop by the invading tumour. Ultrasonography or CT scanning may show the pancreatic mass and the dilated biliary tract. Pancreatic scintiscans with selenomethionine can be useful, but too many scans are falsely abnormal (false positive) and so less are now performed. Transhepatic or retrograde cholangiography will demonstrate the bile duct obstruction, and retrograde pancreatography will reveal the distorted or blocked pancreatic duct. Fine needle percutaneous aspiration of the pancreatic tissue is now being carried out, and provides cytological smears. The needle is passed through the anterior abdominal wall and guided by ultrasonography.

However, final diagnosis is often at laparotomy.

168 *Chapter 17*

## Treatment

Treatment is only palliative since, apart from ampullary carcinomata, the tumour can never be fully resected. A cholecyst jejunostomy bypass operation is carried out to relieve the biliary obstruction. If there is duodenal obstruction or if it is likely to develop, then a gastrojejunostomy is also performed to prevent the distressing pyloric stenosis syndrome. A transhepatic or retrograde stent can sometimes be placed to drain the biliary tract, and at present this is reserved for the patient unfit for surgery. Chemotherapy is almost useless and radiotherapy is probably not effective.

The 5 year survival is almost zero, and the majority of patients rapidly deteriorate and die in less than a year.

## PANCREATITIS

Only the biliary features of pancreatitis are described here.

Acute or chronic inflammation of the pancreas with damage to the acini can cause swelling and hardening of the pancreatic head sufficient to obstruct the lower common bile duct. Chronic pancreatitis is difficult to differentiate clinically from carcinoma of the pancreas, sometimes even at surgery, and mistaken cases probably account for the long survival in patients thought to have carcinoma of the pancreas. Biopsy of the pancreas at surgery carries a risk of leak of pancreatic juice, and the histological appearances of the specimen can be difficult to interpret.

Alcohol is the usual cause of chronic pancreatitis. So in a jaundiced patient with pancreatitis, surgery should be carried out only if the jaundice persists for longer than 3–4 weeks during which the patient is kept abstinent, for the swelling often remits.

## Diagnosis

Diagnosis may be helped by a history of prolonged heavy alcohol intake, raised serum amylase levels, sometimes to levels greater than three times the upper limit of normal, and patchy calcification of the pancreas on plain abdominal X-ray, as it crosses the spine at the L1 vertebra.

## Treatment

Total abstinence for life is strongly recommended. If the patient can do so, then the chances of recovery from an episode of jaundice, and of not relapsing later, are greatly increased. Even so many are unable to resist returning to the bottle!

Bypass surgery procedures are similar to those for carcinoma of the pancreas, but are needed less often.

## FURTHER READING

Bismuth H. & Malt R.A. (1979) Carcinoma of the biliary tract. *New England Journal of Medicine* **31**, 704–6.

Classen M. & Schreiber H.W. (eds) (1983) Biliary tract disorders. *Clinics in Gastroenterology* **12**, No 1.

Schoenfield L.J. (1977) *Diseases of the Gall Bladder and Biliary System*. Wiley, New York.

# Chapter 18
# Congenital and Other Lesions
# of the Biliary Tract

## BILIARY ATRESIA

Various degrees of congenital atresia, or maldevelopment of the extrahepatic or intrahepatic biliary tract occur. Other congenital lesions are associated with them.

### Clinical features

Cholestatic jaundice develops a few days after birth, but unlike many other causes of transient neonatal jaundice, it persists. Itching can be severe. At first the child does well, but later growth is retarded and a large liver and spleen follow as a secondary biliary cirrhosis develops (*see* chapter 10). Hypercholesterolaemia occurs with deposits of cholesterol of the skin, i.e. xanthomata. Steatorrhoea due to a shortage of bile acids in the intestine causes malabsorption of fat soluble vitamins and hence biliary rickets due to deficiency of vitamin D.

### Diagnosis

Diagnosis is by percutaneous cholangiography, retrograde cholangiography and by liver biopsy.

Intrahepatic atresia is not a clear-cut condition and overlaps with neonatal hepatitis (*see* chapter 4). Liver biopsy specimens reveal a reduced number of bile ducts in the portal tracts.

### Treatment

Treatment is medical, with vitamins A, D and K and cholestyramine for itching, and for extrahepatic atresia, surgery. In some children there is sufficient common hepatic duct or main intrahepatic ducts to achieve an anastomosis with a loop of intestine. Transplantation of the liver has been performed for this condition with some success.

Extrahepatic atresia causes death from liver failure, bleeding from oesophageal varices, or infection usually by the age of 6 months. Children

## Congenital and other Lesions of the Biliary Tract

with intrahepatic atresia surprisingly survive up to 10 or more years.

## CHOLEDOCHUS CYST

A choledochus cyst is one or more congenital local enlargements of a section of the common bile duct. They may be small or so large that they displace neighbouring organs and its incidence in females predominates. Adenocarcinoma of the bile duct may develop in the cyst.

They usually present in childhood with pain, jaundice and fever. Large cysts are occasionally also palpable. Treatment is by anastomosis of the cyst to the intestine, or resection.

## CONGENITAL DILATATION OF THE BILIARY TRACT

Partial or widespread congenital dilatation of the biliary tract is sometimes called Caroli's disease. It is associated with other congenital lesions, and with congenital hepatitis fibrosis (*see* chapter 10), but is uncommon.

Serious cholangitis and septicaemia are frequent in childhood or later. Transhepatic or retrograde cholangiography will reveal the bizarre and irregular lumen of the ducts. There are often intrahepatic gall stones.

Treatment is conservative, for surgery is often followed by recurrent cholangitis. Carcinoma of the ducts may occur.

## CONGENITAL ABNORMALITIES OF THE GALLBLADDER

Like other organs, there are many types of anatomical abnormality, some rare.

*Absence* of the gallbladder is rare. It is important only in that it confuses when cholecystography or retrograde cholangiography fails to opacify a gallbladder. Gall stones are then suspected, and laparotomy inevitably follows!

*Folded* gallbladders are not uncommon. Various degrees of folding of the fundus or the body occur. Folding of the fundus is sometimes likened to a Phrygian cap, worn by French revolutionaries.

*Intrahepatic gallbladder* is when the gallbladder lies mostly within the liver parenchyma.

## SCLEROSING CHOLANGITIS

With sclerosing cholangitis there is progressive inflammation, fibrosis and stricturing of the intrahepatic and/or extrahepatic bile ducts and gallbladder. It is uncommon. If there is no known aetiology then it is termed *primary*,

172 *Chapter 18*

or it may be *secondary* to the prolonged presence of gall stones in the bile ducts, or may be in association with inflammatory bowel disease (*see* chapter 15). Histologically the fibrosis is difficult to distinguish from bile duct carcinoma (*see* chapter 17).

The patient presents with abnormal liver blood (function) tests or later with relentlessly increasing jaundice. Liver biopsy appearances may show concentric fibrosis around small bile ducts in the portal tracts, some inflammatory cells (pericholangitis) and cholestasis. Percutaneous or retrograde cholangiography shows the beading and stricturing. Eventually the intrahepatic ducts become almost obliterated.

There is no treatment apart from controlling itching with cholestyramine and anabolic steroids, and prescribing fat soluble vitamins. Corticosteroids are often given but are not effective.

Death occurs within a few years from liver failure and infections.

## FURTHER READING

Classen M. & Schreiber H.W. (eds) (1983) Biliary tract disorders. *Clinics in Gastroenterology* **12**, No 1.

Editorial (1976) An unusual cholangitis. (Sclerosing cholangitis) *British Medical Journal* **2**, 1090–1.

Howard E.R. (1982) Extrahepatic biliary atresia. *British Journal of Surgery* **70**, 193–7.

Schoenfield L.J. (1977) *Diseases of the Gall Bladder and Biliary System*. Wiley, New York.

# General Reading

Brunt P.W. (1973) The genetics of liver disease. *Clinics in Gastroenterology* **2**, 615–37.

Brunt P.W., Losowsky M.S. & Read A.E. (1984) *The Liver and Biliary System*. Heinemann, London.

Sherlock S. (1981) *Diseases of the Liver and Biliary System*, 6th ed. Blackwell Scientific Publications, Oxford.

Wright R., Alberti K.G.M.M., Karran S. & Millward-Sadler G.H. (eds) (1979) *Liver and Biliary Disease*. Holt Saunders, Eastbourne.

# Index

abdominal veins 4, 9
abdominal X-ray 59, 60, 77, 99, 168
abscess
  liver *see* liver abscess
  subphrenic *see* subphrenic abscess
acetyl cysteine 104
acholuric jaundice *see* jaundice,
  acholuric
acinus 66
acne 115
acute hepatic necrosis 10
addicts, drug 117
adenine arabinoside 117
adenoma of liver 140
aflatoxin 137
aggression, histological 66
air in biliary tract *see* biliary tract, air
  in albendazole 100
albumin 15, 16, 17, 24, 29, 43, 49, 54,
  70, 77, 82, 109, 112, 128, 131,
  141, 143
alcohol 2, 3, 26, 84, 97, 111, 119–23,
  129, 136, 168
alcoholic 5, 6, 7, 8, 12, 34, 45, 46,
  47, 119, 120
  fatty liver 119–20
  hepatitis 120–1
  liver disease 2, 46, 119–23, 148
alfa-calcidol 46
alkaline phosphatase 20, 53, 77, 81,
  95, 96, 101, 106, 112, 116, 120,
  128, 131, 134, 140, 141, 147,
  152, 153, 154, 158
  isoenzymes 53, 152, 153
alpha$_1$-antitrypsin 5, 111, 128, 129,
  137
alpha-fetoprotein 55, 77, 140

alveolitis, fibrosing 116, 131
*Amanita* 105
amenorrhoea 2, 26, 115
amines 27, 28, 29
amino acids 27, 28
aminotransferases 52, 53, 77, 82, 83,
  95, 104, 106, 107, 112, 116, 128,
  131, 141, 158
ammonium 27, 28, 29
ampulla of Vater 19, 58, 59, 161, 162
amyloidosis 147
anabolic steroids *see* steroids, anabolic
anaesthesia 108
anchovy sauce 96
angioma 64
anorexia 127
antibiotics 106, 109
antidepressant drugs 112
antigen,
  Australian 87
  hepatitis associated (HAA) 87
antimitochondrial antibody
  (AMA) 57, 58, 115, 131
antimony 98, 100
antinuclear factor (ANF) 57, 58, 115,
  132
antithyroid drugs 106
antituberculous drugs 106, 107
aplastic anaemia 82
arteriography, hepatic 59, 62, 140
artery, hepatic 30
arthralgia 80, 86, 115
arthritis 80, 115, 131, 133
*Ascaris* of bile ducts 160
ascites 1, 4, 9, 11, 34, 42, 44, 45, 81,
  100, 116, 120, 127, 131, 140,
  141, 143

# Index

ascorbic acid *see* vitamin C
aspirin 109
asterixis 5, 81
atresia of bile ducts 46, 170-1
  intrahepatic 74, 76, 132, 170-1
  extrahepatic 74, 76, 132, 170-1
auscultation of liver 10
Australian antigen *see* antigen, Australian
autoantibodies 49, 57, 91, 115, 117
autoimmune liver disease 54, 57, 58
azathioprine 116-7

barium swallow/meal 34, 58, 59, 60, 166, 167
bile 13, 16, 18, 19, 20, 23, 46, 53, 60, 71, 72, 74, 135, 156-7, 162
  limey 160
  lithogenic 157
  white 158
bile acids 16, 18, 19, 20, 21, 22, 23, 24, 29, 46, 51, 154, 157, 162, 170
bile ducts 65, 101, 130-1, 170
  atresia *see* atresia of bile ducts
  carcinoma *see* carcinoma of bile ducts
  stricture *see* stricture of bile ducts
bile plugs 19, 20, 83, 106, 151
biliary obstruction *see* cholestasis
biliary stent 61, 165, 168
biliary tract (tree) 58, 59, 60, 61, 63, 64, 99, 132, 164-9, 170-2
  air in 159
  congenital dilatation of 171
bilirubin 13, 14, 15, 16, 17, 18, 20, 24, 49, 50, 68, 77
  conjugated 16, 17, 18, 20, 49, 50, 51, 52, 66, 70, 74, 77, 81, 82
  direct/indirect 49
  unconjugated 16, 17, 18, 50, 51, 66, 69, 70, 71, 72, 77, 156, 157
bilirubin binding 109
bilirubin conjugation 15, 16, 29, 69, 70, 71, 72, 73
biliverdin 13, 14
biopsy, needle
  of liver 61, 64-5, 72, 74, 77, 83, 93, 94, 97, 107, 111, 112, 115,

116, 128, 135, 136, 139, 141, 143, 146, 147, 154, 170, 172
  of pancreas 167, 168
biopsy, transjugular, of liver 65
bithionol 101
blackouts 123
bleeding 93, 116, 131
blistering 149-51
bowel disease, inflammatory 111, 112, 146, 147, 148, 154-5, 172
bridging necrosis 83
bromsulphthalein test 49, 56, 57
bruising 2, 4, 7, 25, 81, 93, 94, 105, 127
bruit 10, 139, 140
Budd-Chiari syndrome *see* syndrome, Budd-Chiari
bush teas 144
bypass, small bowel 148

caeruloplasmin 54, 136
calcification
  of liver 139
  of pancreas 168
calcified gallbladder *see* gallbladder, calcified
calcitriol 46
calcium 47, 157
canaliculus 15, 16, 18, 19, 53, 65, 83, 106, 151
caput medusae 9
carbon tetrachloride 103, 105, 136
carcinoma
  of ampulla of Vater 58, 166-7
  of bile ducts 74, 101, 141, 155, 164-5, 171, 172
  of the gallbladder 161, 164
  of the liver (hepatocellular) 1, 10, 62
  of the pancreas 11, 58, 60, 74, 145, 164, 167-8
  of the stomach 58, 60, 154
cardiac failure 129, 134, 139, 143
cardiomyopathy 123, 125, 133
Caroli's disease 171
carriers of (HBV) 87, 89, 90, 116, 140
Casoni test 99
cells, ground glass 83
cerebellar degeneration 123, 125

# Index

charcoal 104
Charcot's biliary fever 160
chenodeoxycholic (chenic) acid 20, 21, 22, 162
chest X-ray 59
Chinese liver fluke *see* liver fluke, Chinese
chlormethiazole 121
chloroform 28
chloroquine 97, 98
chlorpromazine 107
cholangiocarcinoma *see* carcinoma of bile ducts
cholangiography
  intravenous 59, 61
  percutaneous (transhepatic) 59, 61, 77, 83, 159, 160, 162, 164, 166, 167, 170, 171, 172
  retrograde *see* endoscopic retrograde cholangio-pancreatography
cholangitis 3, 76, 95, 101, 132, 156, 157, 158, 160–1, 171
  chronic destructive non-suppurative *see* cirrhosis, primary biliary
  sclerosing 74, 154, 164, 171–2
cholecystectomy 61, 74, 159, 160, 161, 163
cholecystitis
  acute 1, 158, 159, 161
  chronic 1, 158, 159–60, 161, 164
cholecystjejunostomy 60, 165, 166, 167
cholecystography, oral 59, 60–1, 74, 159, 162, 171
cholecystokinin 19, 60
choledochojejunostomy 165, 166
choledochoscopy 159, 161
cholestasis 8, 19, 24, 26, 46, 47, 53, 74, 76, 80, 82, 83, 105, 106, 120, 129, 131, 141, 151, 153, 154, 158, 159, 170, 172
  drug 105, 107
  extrahepatic 2, 19, 20, 53, 56, 65, 76, 82
  intrahepatic 2, 19, 20, 53, 56, 74, 75, 76, 147
  postoperative 108

cholesterol 18, 19, 20, 22, 23, 24, 56, 162, 170
cholestyramine 47, 131, 151, 153, 170, 172
cholic acid 20, 21, 22
chondrocalcinosis 134
chylomicrons 56
cimetidine 35
cirrhosis 2, 4, 8, 10, 26, 29, 30, 31, 32, 35, 38, 40, 42, 43, 44, 53, 54, 55, 56, 64, 65, 74, 81, 84, 89, 91, 93, 104, 109, 111, 112, 114, 115, 116, 117, 126–38, 140, 143, 148, 151, 154, 155, 156
  active 114
  alcoholic 7, 121–2, 127, 128, 129, 134, 140, 151
  cardiac 137, 143, 144
  cryptogenic 5, 129, 130
  drug induced 136–7
  Laennec's 122, 126
  macronodular 126, 131, 132, 161
  micronodular 122, 126
  portal 126
  primary biliary 5, 47, 54, 56, 57, 58, 111, 127, 128, 129, 130–2, 146
  secondary biliary 128, 129, 132, 158, 161, 170
clearance 68
*Clonorchis* 141
clotting *see* coagulation
clubbing 4, 5, 127, 131
coagulation 7, 25, 34, 61, 62, 65, 120, 131
  intravascular 29
coagulation factors 5, 49, 55, 56, 64
codeine phosphate 24
colestipol 47
colic, biliary 1, 158
colitis 96, 154
coma 81
computed tomography (CT) 59, 63, 140, 159, 167
congenital hepatic fibrosis *see* fibrosis, congenital hepatic
congo red stain 147
conjugation *see* bilirubin, conjugation
conjunctivae, bloodshot 7

# Index

constipation 27
collagen diseases 145
constrictive pericarditis 137, 144
contraceptive pill 32, 140, 143, 145, 153
copper 128, 129, 135–6
corticosteroids 83, 122, 114–7, 120, 129, 137, 139, 147, 172
Courvoisier's law 11, 164
Crigler-Najjar syndromes *see* syndrome, Crigler-Najjar
critical micellar concentration (CMC) 22
Crohn's disease 112, 154
cyanosis 78
cyst
  choledochus 171
  hepatic 53, 64
  hydatid 60, 64, 98–100
cystic duct 19, 61
cytomegalovirus 80, 91

Dane particle 87
delirium tremens 6, 122, 123–4
delta antigen 88
dementia 122, 123, 125
deoxycholic acid 21, 22
desferrioxamine 134
dexamethasone 28
diabetes 26, 115, 133, 134, 148, 167
diaphragm, elevation of 95, 96
diarrhoea 74
diazepam 121
diazo reaction 18, 49, 50
diet
  low fat 83
  low protein 28
  low salt 44
diuretics 27, 29, 39, 44, 45, 144
DNA polymerase ($DNA_p$) 87, 88, 89
doxorubicin 140
drainage of biliary tract 165–6
drug metabolism 26
drugs 3, 79, 103–9, 146
Dupuytren's contracture 4, 5, 119, 127

*Echinococcus* 98
Ehrlich's reagent 17, 49, 50, 51, 76
electroencephalogram 26

embolisation of hepatic artery 62, 139, 140, 142
emetine 97
emphysema 55, 131
empyema 147
  of gallbladder *see* gallbladder, empyema of
encephalopathy
  hepatic 1, 4, 6, 7, 26, 27, 34, 35, 39, 81, 100, 104, 120
  Wernicke's 45, 123
endoscopic retrograde cholangiopancreatography (ERCP) 58, 61, 77, 83, 159, 162–3, 164, 165, 166, 167, 170, 171, 172
endoscopic sphincterotomy 59, 162–3
endoscopy 36, 58–9, 162–3, 166
*Entamoeba* 94, 96
enterohepatic circulation 16, 17, 19, 21, 24, 46, 50, 157
enzyme induction 53
enzymes 49, 51, 69
eosinophilia 99, 101
epileptic fits 6, 120, 121, 123–4
Epping toxin 103, 105
erythema
  of palms *see* liver palms
  of soles 12
erythropoiesis, ineffective 13, 68, 71
exchange transfusion 73

false neurotransmitters 27
fascies 7, 120, 122
*Fasciola* 101
fasting test 72
fatty acids 70
fatty liver 119–20, 122, 128, 137, 147–8, 152, 154
ferrioxamine 135
ferritin 134–5
fetoprotein *see* alpha-fetoprotein
fetor
  ethanolic 4, 7, 120
  hepatic 4, 7, 26, 81, 127
fibrinogen 25
fibrinolysis 25
fibrosis, congenital hepatic 32, 93, 138, 171
fireworks 105

178 *Index*

fistulae 32
flukes *see* liver flukes
folic acid 40, 46, 120, 121, 122
fractures of ribs 124
frusemide 44, 45
fucidin 109
fulminant liver failure *see* liver failure,
 fulminant

galactosaemia 129, 148
galactose 56, 129
gallbladder 4, 9, 11, 19, 59, 60, 61,
 64, 156–60, 164, 167, 171
 calcified 158, 160
 carcinoma of *see* carcinoma of the
  gallbladder
 empyema of 158, 160
 mucocele of 158, 160
 porcelain 158, 160
 strawberry 158, 160
gall stones 1, 2, 11, 19, 59, 60, 64,
 72, 74, 77, 95, 101, 151, 153,
 156–63, 171, 172
 calcified 60, 156, 159, 162
 cholesterol 156–7
 dissolution of 162
 mixed 156–7
 pigment 156–7
gamma globulin 86
gamma glutamyl transferase 52, 77,
 82, 112, 120, 159
gastric erosions 34, 35, 36, 58
gastroscopy 34
giant-cell hepatitis *see* hepatitis,
 giant-cell
Gilbert's syndrome *see* syndrome,
 Gilbert's
glandular fever *see* infective
 mononucleosis
globulins 24
glomerulonephritis 116, 117
glucuronic acid 15, 71
glucuronides (mono- and di-) 15, 16,
 72, 73, 157
glucuronyl transferase 15
glutathione 104
glycogen storage disease 149
gout 123
 *see also* hyperuricaemia

granulomata 94, 100, 106, 146, 147
ground-glass cells *see* cells,
 ground-glass
gumma 94
gynaecomastia 4, 8, 9, 26, 115, 127

haem 13, 14, 15, 68–9
haemangioma
 capillary 139
 cavernous 139
haematemesis 2, 4, 34, 127
haemochromatosis 8, 26, 64, 122,
 129, 132–5, 140
haemoglobinopathies 69, 72
haemoglobinuria, paroxysmal
 nocturnal 143
haemolysis–16, 50, 68–70, 72, 73, 82,
 97, 108, 109, 120, 135, 147, 156
haemophilia 86
haemorrhage, gastrointestinal 27, 34,
 116, 136
haemorrhoids (piles) 4, 12, 36
haemosiderosis 132
hair loss 4, 5, 9, 12, 26
halothane 108
hepatic arteriography *see*
 arteriography, hepatic
hepatic artery *see* embolisation,
 ligation
hepatic coma 6, 26
hepatic encephalopathy *see*
 encephalopathy
hepatic necrosis, acute 5, 104
hepatic veins 17
hepatic venous pressure 30
hepatitis
 active chronic 58, 89, 111, 129
 acute 12, 19, 26, 30, 51, 54, 55, 65,
  74, 76, 90, 91, 93, 94, 111, 152
 acute alcoholic 56, 79, 111, 120–1
 acute viral 3, 77, 79–92
 aggressive 113–4, 131
 bacterial 79, 93–7
 chronic 2, 54, 57, 65, 74, 79, 81,
  84, 89, 91, 93, 109, 111–8
 auto-immune 111, 115, 116, 127,
  128, 130, 145
 drug 79, 103–9, 146
 giant-cell 76

## Index

179

infections 85
lupoid 114
needle-stick 86
neonatal 55, 76, 137, 170
non-A, non-B 90–1, 108, 111, 112, 117
persistent chronic 89, 111, 112–3
serum 86
toxic 103–9
hepatitis A 84, 85–6, 112, 117
hepatitis A antibody (anti-HA) 77, 83, 85–6
hepatitis B 80, 81, 84, 86–90, 108, 111, 112, 114, 117, 137, 152
chronic 88, 116–8, 121, 129
post-transfusion 91, 108
hepatitis B antibodies 88, 89, 90
hepatitis B core antibody (anti-HBc) 115
hepatitis B core antigen (HBcAg) 83, 87, 88, 89, 117
hepatitis B 'e' antigen (HBeAg) 88, 89, 90
hepatitis B surface antigen (HBsAg) 77, 83, 87, 88, 89, 114
hepatitis B vaccine 90, 140
hepatolenticular disease *see* Wilson's disease
hepatoma 44, 55, 63, 89, 117, 123, 133, 140–1, 143
hepatorenal syndromes 28–30, 45
hepatomegaly 1, 4, 8, 10
hepatoxins
  predictable 103–5
  unpredictable 106–9, 111
hepatotropic viruses *see* virus, hepatotropic
herpes simplex 80, 91
hirsutes 115
histocompatibility antigens (HLA) 115, 116, 121
histology 65–6
Hodgkin's disease 147
homosexuals 86, 90, 117
hyaline sclerosis 120
hydatid cyst *see* cyst, hydatid
hyperaldosteronism 43

hyperbilirubinaemia 50, 65–78, 112, 140, 141
  conjugated 2, 74–6, 153
  unconjugated 68–73, 107, 109
  *see also* jaundice
hypercalcaemia 47, 140
hypercholesterolaemia 170
hypersplenism 25, 42, 47, 100
hypoglycaemia 6, 26, 120, 123–4, 140, 149, 152
hypoglycaemic drugs 106
hypokalaemia 27, 44, 45
hyponatraemia 29, 45, 124

icterus neonatorum 73
ileum 21, 24, 151
ileus, gallstone 158, 161
immune globulin 86, 90
immunoglobulins 49, 54, 82, 116, 128, 131, 147
impotence 2, 26
Indian childhood cirrhosis 157
indirect bilirubin 50
ineffective erythropoiesis *see* erythropoiesis, ineffective
infections 27, 29, 47
infectious hepatitis 85
infective mononucleosis 80, 91, 146
inflammatory bowel disease *see* bowel disease, inflammatory
injections 3
insulin 26
interferon 117
intravascular coagulation 25
iron 26, 64, 97, 103, 105, 122, 128, 129, 132–3, 151
  isoniazid 94, 107
itching 2, 5, 20, 47, 76, 116, 127, 131, 132, 153, 170, 172

jaundice 1, 2, 3, 4, 8, 17, 20, 29, 46, 47, 59, 61, 65–78, 79, 80, 81, 85, 91, 93, 94, 95, 96, 97, 99, 104, 105, 106, 107, 108, 111, 115, 116, 117, 122, 127, 128, 130, 132, 136, 140, 141, 143, 147, 148, 152, 153, 154, 158, 159, 161, 164, 166, 167, 171, 172

acholuric  17, 51, 69, 76
  conjugated  56, 74–6
  extrahepatic  51, 68, 74–5
  familial  2
  hepatic (intrahepatic)  51, 68, 70–6
  neonatal  69, 70, 71, 73–4, 137, 170
  obstructive  19, 75
  physiological  70, 73
  posthepatic *see* jaundice,
    extrahepatic
  postoperative  108
  postpump  108
  post transfusion  91, 108
  of pregnancy  74
  prehepatic  68–70
  regurgitant  68
  retention  68
  surgical  75
  unconjugated  68–73, 108, 144
  *see also* hyperbilirubinaemia

Kayser-Fleischer rings  4, 8, 135, 136
kernicterus  16, 17, 69–70, 73
kidney  28, 136
Korsakoff's psychosis  123–4
Kupffer's cells  54, 63, 65, 97, 98, 134
kwashiorkor  148

lactulose  27, 28, 39
laparoscopy  59, 65, 74, 140, 141
lassa fever  80, 91
LE cells  114, 115
lecithin (phosphatidylcholine)  18, 19,
    22, 23, 24, 157
lecithin cholesterol acyl tranferase
    (LCAT)  20
*Leishmania*  98
leishmaniasis  98
*Leptospira*  93
leptospirosis  28, 93–4
lethargy  127, 133
leucopenia  42, 47
libido, loss of  2
ligation of hepatic artery  139, 140
lipids  49, 156
lipoproteins  20, 56, 119, 120
lithocholic acid  21, 22
liver abscess  3, 10, 53, 59, 63, 64,
    94–7

amoebic  94, 96–7
  pyogenic  94–7, 99, 160
liver biopsy *see* biopsy, liver
liver blood (function) tests  49–50,
    52–8, 128
liver (cell) failure  13, 25, 26, 28, 29,
    40, 44, 45, 55, 82, 104, 106,
    107, 108, 126, 131, 134, 143,
    147, 151, 170, 172
liver failure, fulminant  26, 81, 82
liver flap (asterixis)  4, 5, 6, 26, 34,
    81, 127
liver fluke, Chinese  101, 141, 160
liver flukes  100–101
liver metastases  59
liver palms (palmar erythema)  4, 26,
    115, 127, 152
liver scan *see* scan, liver
lobule  65–6, 83, 93, 94, 103, 112
Looser's zones *see* pseudofractures
lupoid hepatitis  114
lupus erythematosis  58, 114, 145
lymphomata  32, 41, 74, 141

macrocytosis  120, 122
malabsorption  24, 25, 55
malaria  97–8
Mallory's hyaline  120
malnutrition  137
mannitol  29
Marburg virus  80, 91
mebendazole  100
melaena  2, 4, 34, 127, 166
meningitis  93, 94
metastases  59, 63, 139, 141–2
methionine  104
methotrexate  129, 136
methyl dopa  109, 129, 137
methysergide  142
metoclopramide  141
metronidazole  97
micelles  16, 18, 19, 22, 23, 24, 46,
    157
  mixed  22
microsomal enzymes  103, 119
monoamine oxidase inhibitors  106,
    107
mononuclear cells, atypical  82
mononucleosis, infective  91, 146

## Index

mucocele of gallbladder *see* gallbladder, mucocele of
Murphy's sign 8, 159, 160
muscle wasting 5, 12, 122, 123, 125, 127
mushroom poisoning 103, 105
myxoedema 73, 131

nails
  clubbed 4, 5, 12
  white 4, 5, 127
necrosis of femoral head 123
necrosis, piecemeal 131–4
needle-stick hepatitis *see* hepatitis, needle-stick
neomycin 28, 39
neonatal hepatitis *see* hepatitis, neonatal
neonatal jaundice *see* jaundice, neonatal
neonates 16, 70, 71, 73, 109, 136
nephritis 94
neuropathy, peripheral 5, 12, 122, 123, 124, 125
nicbofan 101
nicotinamide *see* vitamin $B_2$
nicotinic acid test 72
night blindness 46
niridazole 101
novobiocin 109
nucleotidase 53
nutmeg liver 143
nystagmus 45, 123, 124

obesity 8, 123, 125, 127, 148
obstructive jaundice *see* jaundice, obstructive
oedema 1, 2, 4, 12, 34, 42, 45, 100, 116, 127, 143
oedema, cerebral 28
oesophagogastroduodenoscopy 58
oestrogens 105, 153, 157
osteomalacia 46
osteomyelitis 147
osteoporosis 123
oxymetholone 48
oxyphenisation 109, 137

pain
  biliary 158, 159, 160, 162, 171
  from liver 1, 41, 42, 72, 80, 95, 96, 99, 112, 140, 141, 142, 143, 152, 160
  pancreatic 167
palmar erythema *see* liver palms
palpation of liver 10, 95, 96
pancreas 59, 77, 133
pancreatitis 32, 123, 125, 158, 161, 168
pancreatitis, chronic 74, 123, 125, 168
paper money skin 7
paracentesis 27, 44
paracetamol 103, 104
parasites 97–101
Parentrovite 40, 45
parotid enlargement 7, 122, 127
Paul-Bunnell test 77, 91
penicillamine 132, 136
penicillin 93, 94
peptic ulcer 34
percussion of liver 10, 64, 95
pericholangitis 154–5, 172
peritoneo-venous shunt 44
peritoneum 59, 64, 99, 101
peritonitis 61
Perl's stain 134
pernicious anaemia 71
persistent chronic hepatitis *see* hepatitis, persistent chronic
phenobarbitone 48, 70, 72, 73
phenothiazines 107
phenylbutazone 106
phenytoin 106
phosphorus, yellow 103, 105
photosensitivity 149–51
phototherapy 73
phrygian cap, gallbladder 171
pigmentation 4, 8, 131, 133, 135
plasmapheresis 48, 132
plasma proteins 49, 53
*Plasmodium* 97
platelet count 64, 83
platelets 25
pleural effusion 95, 96
*Pneumoccus* 47
polyarteritis 81, 87, 117, 145

182 *Index*

polycystic disease 28
polycythaemia 32, 120, 140, 143, 145
porcelain gallbladder *see* gallbladder,
    porcelain
porphobilinogen 51, 149–50
porphyria
  acute intermittent 51
  congenital 149–50
  erythropoietic 149–50
  hepatic 122, 133, 149–50
porphyrin 13, 50, 149–50
portal caval shunts *see* shunt, portal
    caval
portal hypertension 2, 9, 11, 30, 31,
    32, 34, 40, 41, 42, 43, 62, 97,
    100, 126, 136, 138, 143
portal hypertension
  intrahepatic 9
  left-sided 32, 144
  postsinusoidal 31, 32, 33
  presinusoidal 31, 32, 33, 41, 42,
    100, 145
portal tracts 20, 30, 65–6, 83, 93,
    112, 113–4, 120, 128, 130, 100,
    146, 147, 170, 172
portal vein *see* vein, portal
portal vein thombrosis 31, 32
post-hepatitis syndrome *see* syndrome,
    post-hepatitis
post-operative jaundice *see* jaundice,
    postoperative
post-transfusion hepatitis *see* hepatitis,
    post-transfusion
praziquantel 101
pregnancy 32, 55, 74, 105, 152–3
primaquine 98
primary biliary cirrhosis *see* cirrhosis,
    primary biliary
proctocolitis, ulcerative 112
protein binding 69–70
protein synthesis 24
prothrombin 25
prothrombin complex factors 2, 5, 55
prothrombin time 35, 47, 55, 64, 77,
    82, 83
protoporphyria 150, 156
pruritis *see* itching
pseudofractures (Looser's zones) 46
psoriasis 136

purpura 4, 25, 94
pyloric stenosis 166, 167
pyridoxine 46

Q fever 80, 91, 146
quinine 98

radiology 59
radiotherapy 139, 140, 164, 165, 167,
    168
ranitidine 35
rashes 80, 87, 117, 136
regeneration nodules 33, 43, 126, 131,
    132
renal dialysis 86, 90
renal failure 29, 93–4, 104, 105, 147,
    152, 160
renal tubular acidosis 116
renal tubular necrosis 30
reticulin condensation 66
reticuloendothelial cells 25, 69, 154
reticuloses 32
rhesus incompatibility 17, 73
rheumatoid arthritis 109, 145, 147
rheumatoid factor 115, 132
riboflavin 45
rickets 46, 170
Riedel's lobe 10
rifampicin 70–1, 94, 107, 109
Rift Valley fever 80, 91
rigors 80, 95, 160
rose bengal dye 63
rub
  hepatic 11, 95, 96, 140
  splenic 11
rubella 76, 80, 91

salicylates 16
sarcoidosis 32, 131, 146–7
scan
  biliary 63
  liver (scintiscan) 42, 59, 63, 77,
    95, 96, 99, 128, 139, 140, 141,
    143
  pancreatic 167
  selenomethionine 59, 63, 167
schistosomiasis 32, 40, 101–101, 126,
    138
scleroderma 131, 145

# Index

sclerosis, endoscopic 34,36, 37, 38, 58, 101, 145
scratch marks 4, 5, 81
secretin 19
sedimentation rate 82
selenomethionine scan *see* scan, selenomethionine
Sengstaken balloon (tube) 34, 36, 37, 40
septicaemia 93, 94
serum hepatitis *see* hepatitis, serum
sex hormones 26
shunt
 peritoneo-venus (Le Veen) 45
 portal caval 27, 38, 39, 40, 41, 42, 101, 145
 Le Veen *see* shunt, peritoneo-venous
 porto-systemic 47, 126, 128
sicca syndrome 116, 131
sickle cell disease 70, 71
sinusoids 15, 31, 33, 42, 62, 63, 65
smooth muscle antibody 57, 58, 115, 132
sodium 43, 44
space of Disse 65, 147
spherocytosis 71
sphincterotomy *see* endoscopic sphincterotomy
spider naevi 4, 7, 26, 115, 120, 122, 127, 151
spirochaetes 93
spironolactone 8, 44, 45
spleen 1, 42, 59, 60, 62, 63, 64, 69, 81
splenectomy 42
splenic notch 11
splenomegaly 4, 9, 10–11, 12, 34, 40, 41, 42, 97, 98, 100, 116, 127, 131, 145, 147, 170
spur cells 120
steatorrhoea 24, 132, 154, 166, 167, 170
steatosis *see* fatty liver
steroids, anabolic 48, 105, 132, 172
stool
 pale 2, 74, 76, 77, 79, 80, 131
 silver 166
storage diseases 32

strawberry gallbladder *see* gallbladder, strawberry
strictures of bile duct 59, 158, 160, 161
subdural haematoma 124
subphrenic abscess 59, 95
sulphonamides 16, 106, 109
surgery, liver and 29, 38
sweating 12
syndrome
 Budd-Chiari 32, 33, 129, 137, 140, 143–4
 Crigler-Najjar 70, 72–3
 Dubin-Johnson 74, 75
 Felty's 145
 Gilbert's 71–2, 73
 post-cholecystectomy 162
 post-hepatitis 81, 82, 84
 Reye's 148
 Rotor 74, 75
 Zieve's 120
syphilis 93–4

tannic acid 103, 105
telangiectases, facial 120, 122, 127
testicular atrophy 9, 26, 123, 125, 127, 133
tetracycline 103, 104, 153
thalassaemia 70, 71, 72, 133
thiamine *see* vitamin $B_1$
thorotrast 139
thrombocytopenia 42, 61, 62, 100, 139
thrombophlebitis migrans 167
thyrotoxicosis 116
tickling test 10
tissue antibodies *see* autoantibodies
toxaemia of pregnancy 152
toxoplasmosis 76
transamines *see* aminotransferases
transaminitis 82
transferases *see* aminotransferases
transferrin 134
transplantation 132, 140, 149, 170
travel 3
trematodes 100–101
tremor 5, 26, 119
tricuspid regurgitation 137, 144
triglycerides 56, 119, 126, 147

184 *Index*

T-tube 163
tuberculosis 12, 44, 47, 94, 146, 147
tumours, carcinoid 142
tumours of liver 53, 55, 65, 74,
139–42, 145
  primary 139–41
  secondary 141–2
turbidity tests 54
typhoid fever 159

ulcers
  duodenal 58
  gastric 58
  peptic 35, 36
ultrasonography 11, 64, 65, 77, 83,
95, 96, 97, 99, 128, 139, 140,
141, 153, 159, 160, 164, 167
uric acid 120
urine 16, 17, 18, 24, 50, 51, 52, 69,
74, 81, 93, 94, 136, 150
16, 17, 50, 51, 52, 69, 74
  dark 2, 74, 76, 79, 80, 81, 107, 131,
153
urobilin 51
urobilinogen 16, 17, 21, 50, 51, 69,
70, 76, 82
ursodeoxycholic acid 22, 162

varices (oesophageal and gastric) 31,
33, 34, 35, 36, 38, 40, 41, 58,
60, 97, 100, 101, 115, 131, 140,
145, 170
vascular bruit *see* bruit
vasopressin 34, 35, 36
vein
  azygous 34
  central 83
  coronary 31, 40
  hepatic 31, 33, 61, 65, 66, 137, 140,
143–4, 145
  hepatic, webs of *see* webs, hepatic
vein
  oesophageal 33
  portal 30, 31, 39, 62, 65, 128,
144–5
  portal, thrombosis of 145

splenic 144
umbilical 144
vena cava, inferior 9, 140, 143, 144
venesection 35, 151
venography
  hepatic 59, 62, 143–4
  splenic 59, 62, 145
veno-occlusive disease 32, 129, 143,
144
vinyl chloride 139
virological tests 49, 85–9
virus
  Epstein-Barr 80, 91
  hepatitis A 78, 79, 84
  hepatitis B 78, 79, 83, 84, 86–90,
116–8, 140
  hepatotropic 79, 80, 84
  hepatitis non-A, non-B 78, 79,
90–91, 184
  *Ricksettia burnetti* 80, 91
vitamin A 46, 47, 132, 170
vitamin $B_1$ (thiamine) 40, 45, 121,
122, 124
vitamin $B_2$ (nicotinamide) 45, 120
vitamin $B_6$ (pyridoxine) 45
vitamin C (ascorbic acid) 40, 45, 46,
121, 122
vitamin D 46–7, 132, 170
vitamin K 25, 34, 35, 47, 55, 56, 82,
128, 132, 141, 153, 159
vitamins
  fat soluble 26, 46, 170, 172
  water soluble 45–6

webs, hepatic vein 32, 143, 144
Weil's disease 93
Wernicke's encephalopathy *see*
encephalopathy, Wernicke's
Whipple's operation 167
Wilson's disease 8, 54, 65, 111, 129,
135–6

xanthelasma 48, 131
xanthomata 4, 20, 56, 127, 131, 170

yellow fever 80, 92

# Lecture Notes on the Liver

This new book of Lecture Notes follows the tradition of the series to provide clinical students with a wide basis of information on the liver. Apart from the classic diseases such as virus hepatitis and cirrhosis, the author also describes how the liver may be affected in non-hepatic disorders, such as pregnancy and inflammatory bowel disease.

## Some other titles from the Lecture Notes series

Barnes
**Lecture Notes on Gynaecology**
5th edn

Bell
**Lecture Notes on Tropical Medicine**
2nd edn

Beresford
**Lecture Notes on Histology**
3rd edn

Brewis
**Lecture Notes on Respiratory Disease**
3rd edn

Candlish
**Lecture Notes on Biochemistry**

Chamberlain
**Lecture Notes on Obstetrics**
5th edn

Draper
**Lecture Notes on Neurology**
6th edn

Duckworth
**Lecture Notes on Orthopaedics and Fractures**
2nd edn

Edmonds & Hughes
**Lecture Notes on Rheumatology**

Elias & Hawkins
**Lecture Notes on Gastroenterology**

Ellis & Calne
**Lecture Notes on General Surgery**
6th edn

Evans & Henderson
**Lecture Notes on Nephrology**

Farmer & Miller
**Lecture Notes on Epidemiology and Community Medicine**
2nd edn

Gee
**Lecture Notes on Forensic Medicine**
4th edn

Grundy
**Lecture Notes on Pharmacology**

Harris
**Lecture Notes on Medicine in General Practice**
2nd edn

Hughes-Jones
**Lecture Notes on Haematology**
4th edn

Reid
**Lecture Notes on Clinical Pharmacology**
2nd edn

Rubenstein & Wayne
**Lecture Notes on Clinical Medicine**
3rd edn

Sims & Hume
**Lecture Notes on Behavioural Sciences**

Solomons
**Lecture Notes on Dermatology**
5th edn

Templeton & Wilson
**Lecture Notes on Trauma**

Thomson & Cotton
**Lecture Notes on Pathology**
3rd edn

Turner & Blackwood
**Lecture Notes on History Taking and Examination**

Waldron
**Lecture Notes on Occupational Medicine**
3rd edn

Whitby, Percy-Robb & Smith
**Lecture Notes on Clinical Chemistry**
3rd edn

Willis
**Lecture Notes on Psychiatry**
6th edn

Yates & Redmond
**Lecture Notes on Accident and Emergency Medicine**

**Blackwell Scientific Publications Ltd**
Osney Mead, Oxford OX2 0EL
8 John Street, London WC1N 2ES
23 Ainslie Place, Edinburgh EH3 6AJ
52 Beacon Street, Boston,
   Massachusetts 02108, USA
667 Lytton Avenue, Palo Alto,
   California 94301, USA
107 Barry Street, Carlton, Victoria 3053,
   Australia

ISBN 0-632-01338-9